Deep Sleep & Rapid Weight Loss Hypnosis

GUIDED MEDITATIONS AND 100 POSITIVE AFFIRMATIONS TO CHANGE YOUR HABITS AND OVERCOMING INSOMNIA, ANXIETY, OVERTHINKING, BURN FAT & LOSE WEIGHT QUICKLY.

Emily Anderson

Download the audiobook version of this book and you will get also the PDF version for FREE!

You can listen to the audiobook and also read the PDF manuscript.

Take the opportunity!

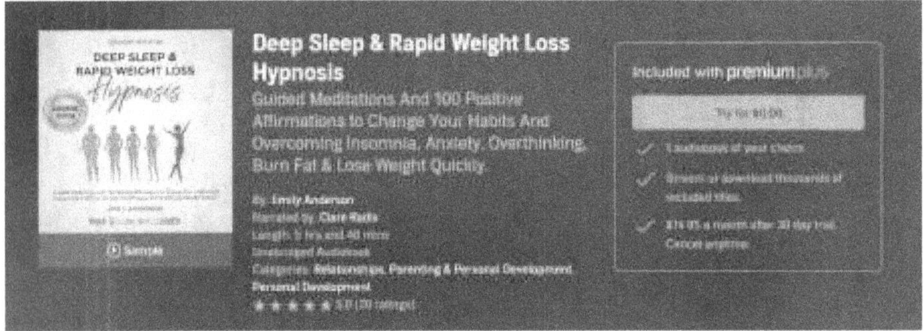

Download it from Audible, typing "Deep Sleep and Rapid Weight Loss Hypnosis Emily Anderson" in the search bar.

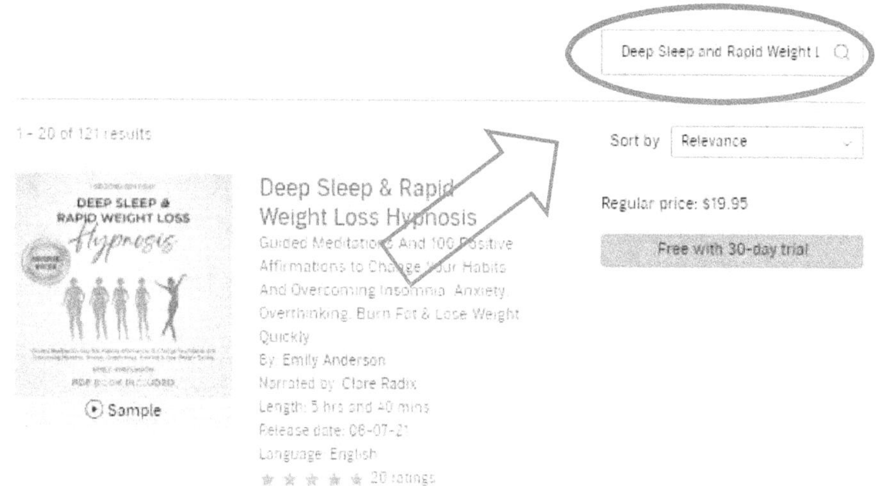

sponsibility or blame be held against the publisher for any reparation, damages, or monetary loss due to the information herein, either directly or indirectly.

Respective authors own all copyrights not held by the publisher.

The information herein is offered for informational purposes solely, and is universal as so. The presentation of the information is without contract or any type of guarantee assurance.
The trademarks that are used are without any consent, and the publication of the trademark is without permission or backing by the trademark owner. All trademarks and brands within this book are for clarifying purposes only and are the owned by the owners themselves, not affiliated with this document

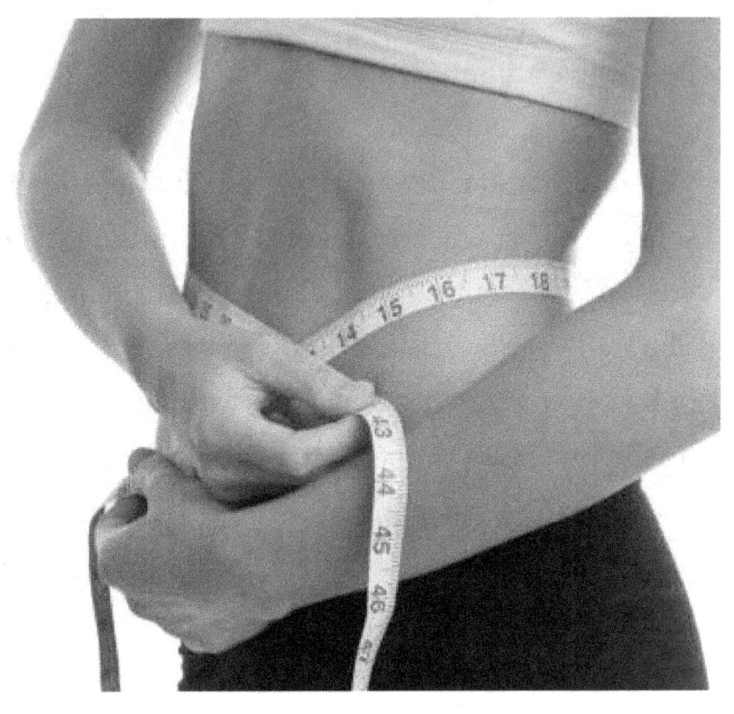

RAPID WEIGHT LOSS HYPNOSIS

HEAL YOUR BODY AND SOUL WITH HYPNOSIS PSYCHOLOGY!

INCLUDES MINI HABITS AND OVER 100 AFFIRMATIONS FOR WOMEN WHO WANT FAT BURN NATURALLY AND STOP SUGAR CRAVINGS.

Emily Anderson

Introduction

Rapid weight loss hypnosis is a way to shed a few extra pounds. But most of the time, it is paired with a diet plan. It is advisable that you continue a good regimen of food, followed by moderate exercise. But, this will allow you to lose weight faster, and if you're a person who has cravings for things, then this will help you immensely. It's also a part of the counseling that some people get. You'll be able to get help on your issues regarding food, and this form of hypnosis will allow you to have a better time with your cravings. You can do this with a professional, but you can also do it on your own. It'll allow you to be in control of your life, and you'll control those bad cravings you have.

When you're using hypnosis, you're in a state of absorption and concentration. You're also in a very relaxed and suggestible state, so whatever is said to you is basically taken in a literal manner. You will use mental images to convey the meaning of the words that are spoken. You'll have your attention focused on that, and when your mind is in a state of concentration, you'll start to have your subconscious handle your cravings. It's a remarkable way to keep yourself in check, and you'll be able to lose a few extra pounds while still trying to keep your body in shape. It's best if you do this with a diet and exercise routine, for it'll allow you to get through it better and achieve more results.

It's best to do this when you have a window of time ready for you to take care of this issue. You'll want at least thirty minutes of quiet time to handle these cravings, ideally an hour at most. You will be handling some pretty substantial matters, so making sure that you're relaxed and able to come back to reality before and after the hypnosis will make it all the better.

The effectiveness varies from person to person. It will help you, and, on average, a person loses about six pounds. You might lose more, but you might not lose as much as expected. If you're trying to lose a ton of weight, this might not help. But, if you're looking to help eliminate cravings in your life and live a healthier lifestyle, then this is definitely the right tool for you. It's a way to help you supplement your exercising plans, and with this, you'll be able to have an even better time when it comes to shedding those pounds fast. There are other benefits of using hypnosis for weight loss. The obvious big one is that you lose weight. That's the one people will notice. You'll start to shed those pounds, and you might lose more than you expected. It won't be significant, such as like fifty pounds or more, but if you want to help your body and allow yourself the benefits of being able to control the cravings to lose weight, then this is perfect for you.

Another benefit that people don't realize is how relaxed you are. You'll actually be able to become more comfortable as a result of this. By relaxing the body, you'll be able also to reduce your blood pressure levels and even stop the risk of heart disease. Hypnosis for weight loss allows you to put yourself in a relaxed state for at least an hour, and when you wake up, you'll feel more comfortable. It can also help with bodily tissues, such as muscle aches and pains. If you want to use this to help with those issues as well, it'll definitely do the trick.

Then there are the lasting benefits of it. These are the benefits that you'll get because of the hypnosis. When you're doing this, you'll be able to tackle those parts of your subconscious that think it's okay to eat when you're stressed, or it'll tell you to eat more than necessary. Sometimes, your mind can be your own worst enemy, and this is undoubtedly one of those times. With hypnosis for weight loss, you'll allow yourself to handle your body in a positive manner. If you do this, you'll actually will enable yourself to control your cravings and desires through the use of hypnosis. It might seem crazy, but it is possible. It's a great way to take life by the horns, and by doing this, you'll be able to allow yourself the benefit of controlling the factors in your life, such as stress or how much you eat, and turning them around to give yourself a more positive image that will benefit you in ways you've never expected before.

If you're the type of person who wants to change your life and your way of thinking to live a healthier life, then hypnosis for weight loss is perfect for you. With this technique, you'll be targeting different parts of the body, and by doing this, you'll be able to have a much better time when it comes to getting rid of the excess weight. It's a great way to lose weight, and by the end of it, you'll be happier, and the scale will look like a friend, instead of an enemy.

Chapter 1 - What is Hypnosis

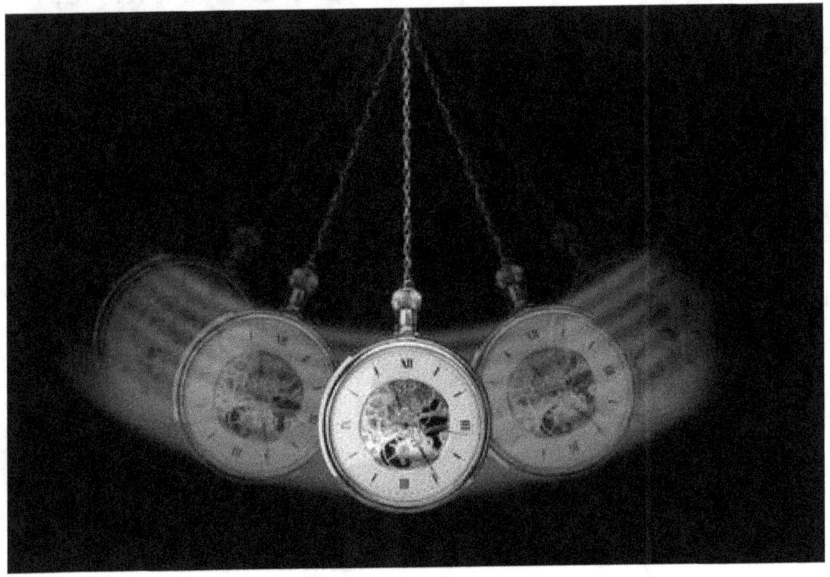

Hypnosis is a state of understanding of focus and concentration. There are two theories about how hypnosis works. The "country" theory implies that subjects enter a different condition of consciousness. The "on-state" concept says that hypnosis isn't an altered state of consciousness. Instead, the topic is responding to a proposal and actively engaging in the semester, Instead of under the control of the hypnotist there are hypnosis methods. Among the very common is that the procedure, which entails keeping a constant stare until the eyes shut at a bright object. You're more when you've entered the state of hypnosis suggestible and more inclined to be more amenable to creating changes. Entering into a trance, relaxed state of consciousness Once a trance, the hypnotist will provide verbal ideas, for example, "if you awaken, you will feel more inspired" or even "you won't drink alcohol." Some argue that hypnosis might help recover repressed memories, treat dependence, cure allergies, and decrease depression and anxiety. Hypnosis is focus and responsiveness to tips. You are inclined to be amenable to creating positive behavioral changes.

We actually enter hypnosis each day without even thinking about it. Hypnosis is not like the things we see in Hollywood. You will not be a mindless drone. Nor will you mindlessly follow absurd commands. Instead, you will be able to use hypnosis to improve learning and to embed new lessons into your subconscious mind. Have you ever said to yourself, "I am going to lose weight"? Yet, a few weeks later you realized that you made that decision but still weighed the same, or even more? This is because you made a decision with the conscious mind, the part that is temporal and acts in the moment, rather than the subconscious mind.

In hypnosis, we are precisely the opposite of what Hollywood portrays. Like in meditation, we are more focused, goal-directed, and intuitively aware. Like an old-time cassette tape, you can record over the messages and the negative behavioral patterns of the past. This is why we will not be giving up anything in this first session. As you add new designs and new lessons to your life, you will naturally and intuitively replace old patterns.

There are several new habits that you will add to your life in this first session. First, you will add food to your diet. You will add nutrient rich foods that are the source of natural energy and health. If you do this each day for a week, you will find that you will effortlessly eat less of the unhealthy things that may have been a part of your life. You will also add a new method of eating. The result will be recording over old patterns that, in the past, have been destructive. You will also add new activities to life and increase your daily physical activity.

The first step is to learn how to enter a state of hypnosis. For beginners, the easiest way to do this is to use guided relaxation. In fact, because guided relaxation is a great way to manage stress, it will be your first new skill for managing weight. Many of our unhealthy patterns come from emotional reactions to stress. Most people never take the time, like you are doing today, to learn how to practice this skill.

So, by going through this necessary process you will have already added a tool that can be useful to you. Relaxation is a way of entering hypnosis because in a relaxed state we are open to new lessons and are comfortable considering new options. There is no right or wrong way to experience this. Begin by getting comfortable in your chair. In a few minutes, you will be very relaxed. However, you will always be attentive, able to hear my voice, and aware of your surroundings. You might listen to outside noises, but these will not distress you. In fact, they will reassure you that you are exactly where you need to be, doing exactly what you need to be doing.

Now that you have found a comfortable place to still the body and the mind, begin by scanning your body. Anywhere you are carrying the tension of the day in your muscles, simply let those muscles relax. Pay attention to the small muscles of the brow and around the eyes. Let them relax as well. Often, tension is held in tissues of the jaw. You can even allow these muscles to relax.

As you relax, notice that you're breathing becomes slower and more natural. As you listen to the quiet in the room or hear the distant sounds of others outside of the room, give yourself permission to enjoy this time of developing a sense of deep relaxation.

As your hands rest on your lap, let them feel very relaxed, very heavy, and very calm. Again, scan your body and relinquish any remaining tension. Relax any residual tension held in the shoulders, back, or legs. Now, notice that your breathing is slower and calm. In just a few moments, your heart rate has even slowed.

This necessary process of physical relaxation can also be used to still the mind. Do not worry if your account has been wandering or thinking. After all, this is what brains do. Imagine yourself under a clear blue sky. You can imagine that you are in a place you have been to before, would like to go, or a situation entirely of your own creation. In the sky, there is a single white puffy cloud, gently drifting towards the horizon. As it floats, send all of your thoughts, cares, and concerns into that cloud. Watch the cloud move farther and farther towards the horizon, until it disappears all together. Now, both your body and mind are completely relaxed. If any other thoughts surface, just allow them to drift towards the horizon after that puffy cloud.

In this state of hypnosis, I am going to give you some direct suggestions. These are not suggestions that come from me, instead they are suggestions you have asked me to make by participating in this session. I am also going to share what are called indirect tips to help you to learn intuitively. I know you have a strong sense of what is right for you, because people who participate in these types of sessions usually do. As a result, learning intuitively will be easy for both your conscious and subconscious mind. The direct suggestions I am going to make will add to your life. I will also share with you some of my own personal experiences, for the path you are on is well-worn.

It is incredible how easy it is for someone to lose weight by adding something into their life, even by adding more food. By adding nutrient dense foods into your diet, your body will naturally and effortlessly respond in ways that are best for it. So by inserting something into your life each day, you will be well on your way to a slimmer, lighter, and healthier you.

The first addition will be adding one pound of fruit and one pound of vegetables to your diet each day. It is incredible how by cutting up a bowl of fruit and a bowl of vegetables, one begins to crave health. Many who have done this have had that much experience. By adding a pound of fruit and a pound of vegetables into your diet each day, you will be just like the others who have made this beneficial change to their lives.

I grew up in Chicago and I remember, as a child, driving with my grandmother to Great Lakes Navel training station. While we were there, we would go to the PX to do our grocery shopping. Each week, on what I assume was my grandfather's payday, we would shop for groceries. My grandmother would cut coupons for our weekly shopping ritual. I remember how long it took to shop and how many bags my grandmother would buy. When we got home, I would help her put the groceries away. We stored some in the kitchen and some in the deep freezer in our garage. I spent the rest of my adult life shopping the way I learned to shop with my grandmother, by making a weekly visit to the store and coming home with a week's supply of groceries.

In 2004, I spent a great deal of time overseas. I had an opportunity to travel to Eastern Europe and to Asia, where I spent my time with local families rather than merely exploring as a tourist. In almost every place I visited on three different continents, the people shopped the same way for food. In every home I stayed in, the families went shopping each day for a small amount of groceries. While walking home in the afternoons, we bought for dinner. We always selected fresh foods, fruits, and vegetables. We usually only purchased the quantity that we would need for that night. It seemed like we were still in the express lane, choosing a few items in a basket and checking out quickly, rather than shopping for a hundred questions to last a week.

And, I noticed a difference. When I began shopping each day, the food was fresh and there was no need to purchase frozen prepared foods, which are usually processed and unhealthy. And so, I began to shop in this new way even upon my return to America. Each day, I stop at the market by my house, usually buying fruit for the next day and a few items for dinner that night. You will also find great benefit in adding a trip to the supermarket in your daily routine and choosing a limited amount of food on each trip. Simply, purchase enough to last for the next day or two.

Chapter 2 - What is Self-hypnosis

The only significant difference between hypnosis and self-hypnosis is that in the first one the operator and the subject are two different people, while in self-hypnosis the operator and the subject coincide in the same person.

It can be very positive to share the self-hypnosis learning experience with another person using the methods described in this book. This shared experience can be of great value to both, as it will unite them mentally and emotionally and promote love and mutual respect.

It is also a fact that learning is more comfortable and faster when done with another person.

Ask your partner to hypnotize you using a procedure similar to the one we used in the second session. Then practice the self-hypnosis exercise for a few days. Ask your partner once again to hypnotize you and reinforce hypnotic suggestion. Practice it again.

The number of times it is necessary to reinforce the procedure depends entirely on you. If you practice the daily self-hypnosis exercise, one or two reinforcement sessions will be sufficient.

But what about those who have no one with whom to share the learning experience of self-hypnosis? What can they do? How can they learn?

Leave your worries aside.

It is possible to use self-hypnosis to solve virtually any type of problem and also to broaden your consciousness and connect with your innate superior intelligence and creative ability. By using self-hypnosis for the latter purpose, hypnosis can be transformed into a meditation.

Self-hypnosis can also be used in those moments when you feel the need for a higher power to intervene in some situation; then it becomes a prayer. The subtle differences between these forms of self-hypnosis lies in the way thoughts are guided once the state of consciousness itself has been altered, that is, when the alpha state has been reached.

Then I will tell you a fun experience that happened to me with self-hypnosis. I had an appointment with the dentist to have two molars removed. Last night I had conditioned myself to stop the flow of blood.

The day of the appointment, when sitting in the dentist's chair, I self-reported. When the dentist removed the teeth, I blocked the flow of blood so that it did not flow through the open wound.

The dentist was perplexed and kept telling his assistant: «It doesn't bleed.

How is it possible? I don't understand it. I smiled mentally, since I couldn't physically smile because of all the devices, cotton and other objects that held my mouth. In addition, I visualized a quick and complete healing. After seventy-two hours the swelling had subsided and the wounds had healed completely;

And now I will tell you another funny experience that one of my patients had with self-hypnosis.

He was part of a group that participated in an investigation about dreams at the local hospital. Once a week my patient slept in the hospital with an electroencephalogram (EEG) connected to his head. This was intended to record the waves of their brain activity.

By observing the graph, doctors could establish if they were in alpha, beta, tit or delta state, and they could also state when the patient was sleeping and when he was awake. My client immediately hypnotized himself as soon as he was connected to the EEG.

The apparatus recorded a deep alpha state, indicative that the subject was sleeping, although he was fully awake. One of the doctors asked: "What's going on here?" Then the man alternately returned to the beta state, then to alpha, then again to beta and finally to alpha while the machine registered it.

The changes confused the doctors until the subject told them what he was doing. The response of the doctors cannot be reproduced here.

I have devised and written practically all the contents of this book in an alpha state. What does this mean? It means that it is possible to develop an activity and keep your eyes open even if one is in an altered state of consciousness. Think about it for a moment.

What a fantastic tool is self-hypnosis! It transports us to another state while we are comfortably and quietly sitting with our eyes closed thinking about a particular objective. But using self-hypnosis in this sense is not easy to achieve since it requires a prolonged period of preconditioning in a hypnotic or auto hypnotic state. Such preconditioning is similar to that used for diet control, but the indications are different; it will be necessary to devise the techniques and suggestions for this case.

And it also requires practice, a lot of practice. Do not forget my words, time and effort will be rewarded with the results. Develop your own discipline and stick to it; the results will be a real success.

It has been proven lately that hypnotism has an impact on the brain which can be measured scientifically.

Doctors from Stanford University had scanned the brains of some volunteers who were told that they were looking at colored objects. The fact was that the objectives were actually black and white.

A scan of their head revealed that the areas of the brain, that used to register color, had increased blood flow. This indicated that these volunteers genuinely 'saw' colors in their eyes of the mind.

There has been more research in this field where in one study, the volunteers were hypnotized with the visualizations of playing tennis, while in reality they were just lying inside the scanning machine. The areas of brain which would have been functional while actually playing tennis were showing increased blood flow in the brain scans. This clearly indicates that our brain cannot distinguish between what actually happens and what it imagines over a prolonged interval of time.

Well, it can be said with firm support of scientific evidence that this "inability of the brain to distinguish between a real experience and hypnotically imagined experience" has tremendous benefits for humans. It thus confirms that professional hypnotists are scientifically sound in claiming that hypnotism has a profound effect on the functioning of our mind, as well as our body.

So, hypnosis can be used for many kinds of physical symptoms and diseases which are mostly due to the psychological component of the mind. Let's take the example of pain control. You sometimes get a cut in your finger while cutting fruits or vegetables with a sharp knife. It hardly registers in your mind. It is only after you look at the blood oozing out of your finger that you start to experience pain. Thus, we can reprogram our brain to imagine that there was no cut, no blood and no pain in any part of your limb and that your arm is feeling superfine and relaxed. This is the information that would be delivered to your mind and you would start getting better under the effect of natural healing mechanisms which work best when you are relaxed in your account.

It is a clear fact in scientific community that positive thinking rewires your brain and so do the positive suggestions during hypnosis. When you feed your mind with positive ideas about achieving something or with visualizations of having something already accomplished, structural changes take place in your brain. These structural changes begin to help you transmute the suggested/imagined experience into its physical equivalent. You see things and opportunities which you never had seen before. You start to find that every situation of your life is in a constant process of helping you. Your goals seem coming to you rather than you going towards them. Your all fears are gone. Your bad habits seem to be leaving you and you start living the life you imagined. Such is the effect of hypnosis.

Chapter 3 - How Does the Mind Work?

Do you want to lose weight? If you are reading this book, your conscious response is probably 'yes'. But what is the answer of your subconscious? If you experience weight loss, it is because your subconscious collaborates well with your inner self. In case of a negative reply, you would doubt whether every part of you wants to go in the same direction. It often happens that the conscious and subconscious mind don't speak the same language. For this reason, it is essential to harmonize all parts of your brain and give them the same command. How can you do it?

Imagine writing a manual for a car that deals eloquently with the body, comfort level, style, color, safety and acceleration features of the car, without saying a word about how its internal engine operates. Could you repair your vehicle if something breaks down while relying on such a description? Clearly not, in the case of machines, we are lucky because we can take the car to a workshop where somebody does comprehend the functions of the engines and can repair it. But what to do when it comes to fixing our minds? We can go to a psychologist for advice, but it is eventually our duty to get our minds right. All our behaviors, constructive or destructive, can be modified by our thoughts. If we learn the nature of our thought system, we find the very secrets of human psychology. The gate to our freedom opens before us as soon as we expose ourselves to the sunlight of purity and wisdom with the right knowledge and comprehension of the functions of our minds. The very first step is to understand how the brain and human consciousness work in general.

How does our inner consciousness work?

We traditionally divide the human mind into two parts: the conscious and the subconscious mind. Conscious functions include analytical thinking, logic, reflection, reasoning and judgmental abilities, short-term memory. The subconscious commands our biological systems, handles response, emotions and long-term memory. While the conscious mind's terrain is only 10%, the subconscious mind occupies 90% of our brain. Therefore, you should keep in mind that the only way to change your life is to learn to command your account at a subconscious level.

What should we know about the subconscious mind?

The subconscious mind always follows our instructions. What does this mean? It means we are in trouble if we do not program it in our favor, and we can reap the rewards if we give the right commands. It will receive the inputs and realize what is reinforced by our emotions. The subconscious mind is an excellent servant but a terrible master. Everything, whether wanted or not, is accomplished once we have accepted the related emotions. The stronger the feelings we recognize, the more effectively and promptly we can achieve a goal. How does it work? We create a thought, the thought creates an image, an image creates emotion, and the feeling creates a reality. We process first through our creative manager, in order for the conscious mind to create a thought. It means that we have the keys to open the gate to the subconscious mind, the executive manager. So, we can learn how to control our thoughts, in order to manage our emotions (Tracy, n. d.).

Sadly, beginning from our childhood, it is inculcated into us that we have to listen to, say and even think, what we do not want, instead of concentrating on what we do want. When you aren't feeling well, what do you usually think, "I do not want to be sick" or "I want to be healthy"? Unfortunately, we very often tend to bring the first sentence into our mind; however, in this case, we put the focus on sickness and not fitness. As you pronounce or think of a word, it already forms a picture in your head. And we know that mental images generate emotions, even strong emotions in us. Let's do a mini exercise. For this, I will ask you not to imagine a specific object! Are you in? OK! So, don't believe a blue apple. What did your mind do immediately? It imagined precisely that: a blue crab. Why? Because as soon as you say the word, the image appears immediately, as the mind does not understand the negations. The negative name cannot be displayed in a picture. Thirdly, if you want to program something in your brain, pay attention to imagining the related scene in the present or in the past, because if your picture takes place in the future, your subconscious mind will think it is only a future project; therefore it wants to realize it only someday in the future. If your subconscious feels the urgency of a project, the realization process will be shorter.

Therefore we have to convince our creative manager to give the right command to the executive manager. To accomplish this task, we need to understand what to focus on with our thoughts simply because we acquire what our thoughts are directed to. It is fundamental to comprehend this simple equation. What you pay attention to now, will return to you in the future. The only thing you need to do is to preserve and nurture it because these thoughts are the creators of your future. If you center on what bothers you, even if you don't want it to be realized, you will have to meet it in the future. Have you ever happened to face the difficulty that you were afraid of? I am sure your answer is affirmative. This is because many times, we experience the fate we want to avoid.

Chapter 4 - Hypnosis and Weight Loss

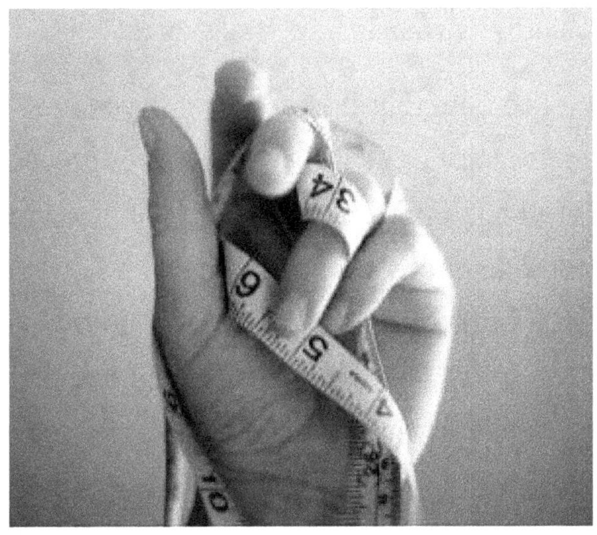

Obesity is rising rapidly in the world and is becoming one of the most significant problems for the urban population. Individuals do all kinds of things, mainly physical workouts, to lose weight, but only a small portion takes nutritious foods into account. Over time most people are used to these patterns, which makes the fight much harder to lose weight. Here weight loss with hypnosis is beneficial, but conclusive findings have not been confirmed scientifically.

First of all, weight loss by hypnosis is not immediate but happens after a person has changed his / her ideas and habits. Therefore, a person begins to lose weight. Hypnotherapists mix images, thoughts, and words and bring them to the mind of a person in order to change the body's picture, perception, and belief. A person is thus prepared to adopt healthy habits to lose weight. Hypnosis can only be used to lose weight if this is done together with other strategies, such as exercise.

It is important to note that it is not for everybody to lose weight using the hypnosis process. To be open to this process, you must be prepared to be hypnotized. Secondly, you need to have complete faith in the hypnotherapist and the techniques used. If you are unable to submit your mind to the guidance of hypnotherapists, it may be a waste of time to undertake the procedure. Besides hypnosis, binaural and isochoric beats may be used to help them lose weight. These beats help reprogram the subconscious mind with frequencies of 4-8 Hz that activate the Theta state of mind.

This state corresponds to a profound trance and is easily achieved by skilled mediators. Monaural beats are also instrumental in weight loss, but most people say isochoric tones are much more useful. Such types of brainwave training mainly influence a person's general health over their weight to alter his or her mind. By changing the emphasis from weight loss to wellbeing, the approach begins to change one to a better mental status that benefits from the fact that it attracts the like. If a person concentrates on the negative aspects of weight loss, he attracts more people than he needs.

Hypnosis, also known as hypnotherapy, refers to the profoundly relaxed, almost transitory state of people. Although people are far more open to suggestions in this society.

When an individual is hypnotized, he is exceptionally calm. You can focus more quickly than "wake up" and consider constructive ideas that enter the subconscious mind. Such suggestions are useful if the person is awake.

A reliable therapist takes the patient time. They're going to communicate with them. And the therapist can try to communicate with the client in the subconscious while the client becomes hypnotized. The psychiatrist would be just like an investigator who tries to find the underlying factor that triggers abuse or unethical behavior.

Using binaural beats, which have been clinically proved to work for everyone, one should concentrate on positive aspects of body health. As a result, you gain better health and ultimately meet other healthier bodies. The use of binaural weight loss beats is much simpler and faster than different approaches, such as food plans and weight loss pills. Of course, other things do need to be done to do so, but binaural beats make the procedure much simpler and more pleasant compared to weight loss in hypnosis.

Hypnosis is a method that is to make suggestions to the hypnotized person placed into an altered state of mind with the intention of ringing in the positive changes in their thought and behavior. If the hypnotized person regains consciousness, he or she may continue to act on your subconscious mind's suggestions, while hypnotized.

This is standard practice for a therapist to communicate with the subconscious mind of the patient to attempt to determine the underlying factors behind the patient's abuse. When you have trouble maintaining optimal body weight, try using hypnosis weight loss. In the conscious state, which has challenging time security from overeating, you'll try, but in his attempt to lose weight, he'll soon overcome the best intentions and fail.

In such cases, you must seriously consider weight loss by hypnosis and be able to fight at will without your conscious mind rejecting their efforts. Everything that means losing weight by hypnosis is pushing optimistic thoughts into the subconscious mind instead of doing it consciously. Weight reduction by anesthesia has a higher chance of success as they change their work culture from the inside out, and reprogramming the subconscious mind will change things for the better, with less brain-conscious resistance.

Using weight loss by hypnosis, you can find that after a diet once appeared challenging to maintain, and the explanation for this change for the better is that the relationship with food has undergone a dramatic shift-without ever knowing its-consciously.

We soon realize that weight loss by hypnosis has made it possible to lead a healthier life and will not find it challenging to make the right choices about a balanced diet. Yeah, he'll also get great pleasure and happiness from his new thinking. Moreover, when the brain sends signals to rescheduling the body's commands, you can even notice changes (positive) happening at the cellular level.

Weight-control hypnosis had also worked when other, more traditional weight-loss methods failed. It can also gain a benefit when coping with weight loss by hypnosis as destroying the cravings to overeat, feeling a strong sense of self-empowerment, improving self-esteem, giving you a more positive image, reducing stress levels and finally finding out what caused you to overeat first.

Hypnosis weight loss, is that a fact? Is that all a bunch of lies? Will people really believe that you can actually extract fat from your body through a method that is as controversial as hypnosis? Okay, believe it or no, many studies have shown the efficacy and truthfulness of this technique and, while weight loss due to hypnosis does not work for everyone in the world, it certainly worth your time because it has been beneficial for thousands of people.

You see, all the temperament is hypnosis. If you can change someone's ability to do it (or avoid doing it in this respect), can you finally change their way of living? That's a reality, and hypnosis means that you can alter how someone behaves or even thinks. And here's where hypnosis weight loss comes into play; actually, it's not that hard to change people's thoughts into healthier people, and hypnosis is based directly on people's sub consciousness, programming their weight loss behavior is natural.

However, this method only works for people willing to be hypnotized. There are plenty of people out there for whom hypnosis is entirely ineffective, primarily due to their thought and impermeability to their values and beliefs. If you're such a person, then weight loss by hypnosis would be an excellent failure, but if you're open to new ideas and strategies, your mind may be sensitive to anesthesia, and you could start losing enormous amounts of weight after hypnotizing.

Bear in mind that weight loss by hypnosis extends to several different places to tackle the issue, it's not because you're going to lose this weight miraculously, it means you're going actually to want to pursue a weight loss program, and that your willpower will be significantly improved, helping you to stick on the weight loss path without feeling the temptation to drop out.

It is also important to remember that if you want to pursue a weight loss through the hypnosis system, you consider all the implications this might have. You must invite an outsider into the depths of your mind and give him permission to reprogram the very principles of life you have created in your life. This doesn't necessarily mean something negative, but it's essential to take note of that before you attempt to sign up for a weight loss by hypnosis program.

Chapter 5 - The Benefits of Having a Healthy Body

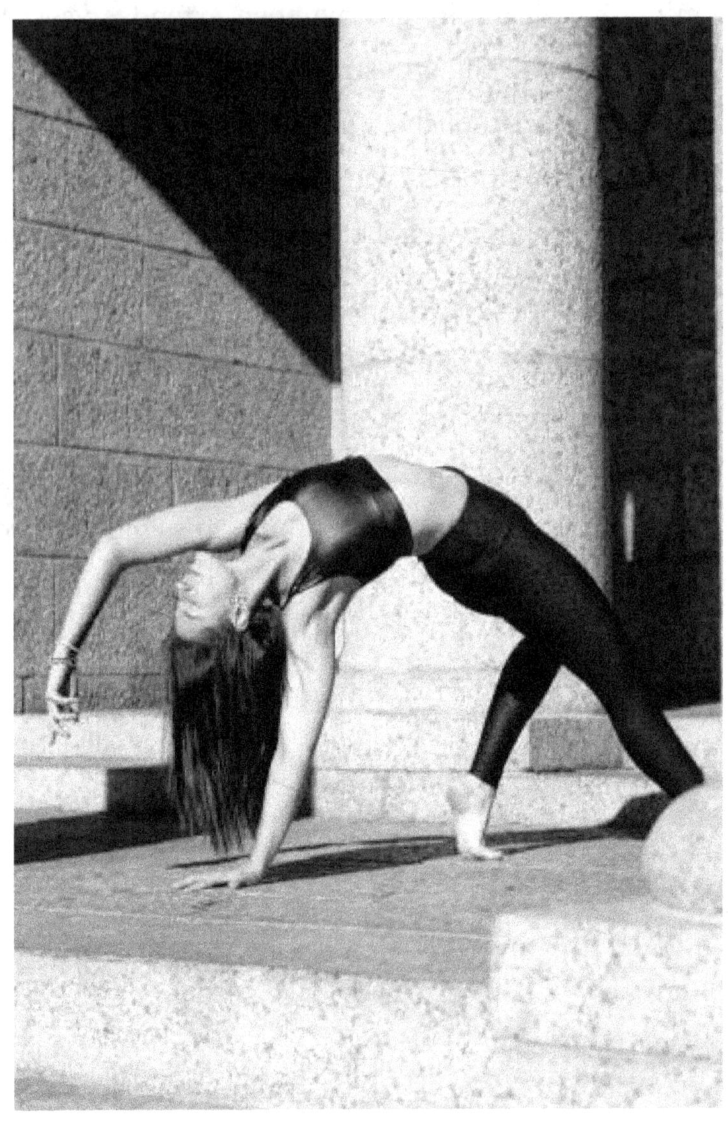

It is crucial to maintain a healthy body to preserve achieves a healthy life. A healthy body enables one to lead an active and more productive life, which directly translates to great achievements and also age gracefully. To maintain a healthy body, one has to have a healthy diet, subject himself/herself to regular exercises, maintain a stress-free mind, have a quality sleep and also, lead a healthy lifestyle. The following are ten important reasons for maintaining a healthy body.

1. Boosts the immune system

A healthy body means that all the body processes are working at their best, and therefore all required antibodies for fighting illness are produced in enough amounts. This way, the body can fight off illnesses and protect the body from getting sick. Even though the body cannot fight off all illness, a healthy body is likely to fight off most seasonal illnesses compared to the non-healthy body. It is advised, however, that if the body's immune system goes down, it is important to avoid consuming alcohol or taking in food and drinks that are sugary as microbes have a high affinity for sugar.

2. Reduces chances of getting any type of cancer

From a biological explanation, cancer is the uncontrolled division of cells due to a mutation of the DNA within cells. DNA is responsible for giving cells instruction on when to divide, how much cells to divide, and also repair cells that need repairing.

When the DNA mutates, the cells divide uncontrollably and not perform the required tasks leading to cancer. Causes of DNA mutations are either inherited genetically, biologically predisposed through chemical causing cancer or unhealthy lifestyles like poor diet, smoking, consumption of loads amounts of alcohol, and obesity. Unhealthy lifestyles are the number one cause of cancer. A healthy body contains a normal DNA, which means a controlled cell division and also, proper repair of cells. It is therefore important to maintain a healthy body

3. Increases the body energy level

A healthy body has high levels of energy, which are as a result of the work put in to achieve it. Being healthy means having a healthy diet. A healthy diet means that the body is supplied with the required vitamins, carbohydrates, and proteins required. Exercising makes the body adapt to harsh treatment. In return, every exercise session leaves the body even stronger than it was before. Enough sleep clears the mind and also gets rid of fatigue. This compilation ultimately translates to the body having high energy levels and more productive.

4. Reduces chances of being infertile

Being overweight or underweight can increase one chance of being infertile. Also, the abuse of recreational drugs and smoking can contribute greatly to infertility. Being overweight, smoking and consuming loads of alcohol in men reduce the sperm count leading to infertility. Both being underweight and overweight in women also contributes to infertility. All the above stated problems are a result of an unhealthy body. Therefore, eating healthy to avoid underweight, exercising to curb obesity and overweight cases and leading a healthy lifestyle and minting a healthy body can go a long way in the cure for infertility.

5. Prevents stroke and heart related problems

Stroke is where the brain is deprived of oxygen for a while, causing death to its cells. Deprivation of oxygen may be caused by blockage of arteries or rupturing of arteries leading to leakage of oxygenated blood responsible for keeping cells up and running. Among the causes of blocked arteries is due to deposition of fat blocking the proper flow of blood to the brain. Other causes may include unhealthy lifestyles and stress. Heart problems include heart attack and coronary artery disease.

Similarly, coronary artery disease is caused by too much cholesterol blocking the supply of blood to the body. A heart attack is the rapture of the coronary artery; it is as a result of the heart pumping blood at a higher rhythmic pressure than the normal one. This creates pressure on the artery causing them to rapture. The best treatment approved by doctors for both diseases is exercising, leading a healthy lifestyle, having enough rest, avoiding stress and also adopting a healthy diet. Doctors stress keeping our bodies healthy as we can fight off illnesses like heart problems and stroke among others.

6. Enhances some career choices

Careers like athletics require athletes to maintain healthy living standards and impressive body physique. Athletes are required to adopt a strict diet, exercise regularly, and subject their bodies to enough sleep and, most of all, avoid consumption of recreational drugs as well as too much alcohol if not a small amount. In the entertainment industry too, models and dancers mostly are required to adhere to similar living standards. These healthy standards ensure their bodies are at optimum health and they can remain top of their careers.

7. Improves longevity

Study within time has shown that having a healthy body ensures one to achieve a long life. Exercising as little as twenty minutes a day reduced the chances of one suffering a premature death. Healthy adjustments like proper diet are also essential in achieving a long life. The healthy body even at an older age also means that one can carry out tasks which would have been hard if they were unhealthy or dead. It also means that one can enjoy more time with family. Grandparents get a chance to see and bond with their grandchildren all because of maintaining their bodies at healthy levels

8.   Helps control body weight

A healthy body is a state acquired after proper care of the body and exercises. Even without trying to lose weight, healthy living standards will ultimately lead to a healthy body weight. A weekly schedule of a few hours of exercise and eating right will go a long way in maintaining a healthy body weight. The body will have a strong immune system, prevent heart diseases and also spike the body energy level all as a result of a healthy body

9.   Improves moods and feelings

A study has proven that exercising our body leaves our bodies relaxed and happy also. This is a result of the release of brain cell chemicals called endorphins. Exercising also ensures that one achieves an athletic physique, which means that one will have improved physical appearances leading to improved self-confidence. We live in a world of constant disappointments and tragedies. It is important to keep out bodies at most health for improved emotional balance and also maximum cognitive functions

10.   Helps manage diabetes

There are two main types of diabetes, type one where the body insulin producing cells are attacked by the body itself. One has to live on insulin shots all his/ her life and type two diabetes where the body is unable to absorb the sugar in the blood and convert it into energy for the cells. Type one diabetes is a result of poor health living standards, lack of exercises and having a poor diet. Early stages of diabetes like Pre diabetes and also gestational diabetes can be controlled by a proper diet and exercise. Maintaining a healthy body will mean that the body will be able to control body insulin balance and reduce fatalities caused by Diabetes like blood pressure, heart attack, kidney failure and hardening of blood vessels

11. Improves the brains memory

A healthy body constitutes a healthy diet; a healthy diet comprises of all the food nutrients. Among these nutrients are vitamins. Vitamins preferably C, E, D, Omega 3, fatty acids and flavonoids are essential in developing a brain with a good memory. A healthy diet also helps fight off dementia and decline of cognitive functions. Dementia is the loss of memory, effects on the ability to speak, think or even solve a problem. Eating healthy will help reduce dementia that which is not caused by physical injury on the brain.

12. Strengthens both the bones and the teeth.

Maintaining a healthy body helps improve the strength of teeth and bones. It is advisable to consume dairy products for calcium three portions a day. One is also required to subject the body to physical exercises, and the most preferred one is lifting weights. A proper diet is essential as well. One is required to consume meals rich in calcium and magnesium for stronger teeth and bones. Many kinds of cereal contain calcium while magnesium is abundantly found in legumes, nuts, whole grains and seeds

13. Boosts self-esteem

Among reasons for having low self-esteem is having an unhealthy body. We live in a world of diversity and one that is rich in different tastes in fashion. Often everyone wants to look good, but at times our bodies often fail us, and this can be bad for our self-esteem. However, this can be changed, and our esteem boosted within no time. A proper diet would be a good start accompanied by regular body exercises and maintaining a healthy mind through rest and controlling what we think. Results take time, but eventually, one achieves a healthy body. This is more like killing two birds with one stone as one can boost their self-confidence by enhancing appearances and also achieve a state of a healthy body through having a healthy body.

14. A Healthy body improves better sleep

Often people with unhealthy bodies go through a lot of difficulties when sleeping. They often sweat a lot in cases of obesity and even find difficulties breathing when asleep. Healthy people sleep well and find no difficulties breathing when sleeping. Subjecting the body to exercises ensures the body process work right, and it burns off excess fats causing sweating during the night. Eating right and avoiding abuse of drugs and alcohol also helps achieve a healthy body. A healthy body, in turn, leads to sound sleep

15. Improves sex life in couples.

Sex is a physical act; it is therefore required for both partners to be physically fit to have a good time. More often than not, once one of the partners gains an unreasonable amount of weight or both of the partners, they start experiencing bedroom problems. Sex is a significant aspect of all couples. If problems arise in this area, the likelihood of separation is high. It is therefore advised of couples that they maintain healthy bodies to avoid bedroom problems.

16. Improves chances of surviving disasters and violence

We live in the 21st century, where the world is a subject of natural disasters as well as man inflicted violence's from robbery to wars. The world is no longer a safe place, and no one is an exemption to this bitter truth. So, in case of an onset of such misfortunes, human beings are supposed to find ways to survive. Among ways of improving chances of survival in such cases is having a healthy body, both strong and athletic. The rule of life would take course and the strong and fit that is those that are healthy are going to survive. A healthy person is more likely to evade himself/herself from a scene of violence by moving away as quickly as possible. An unhealthy person might not be so lucky.

Chapter 6 - Psychology of Weight Loss

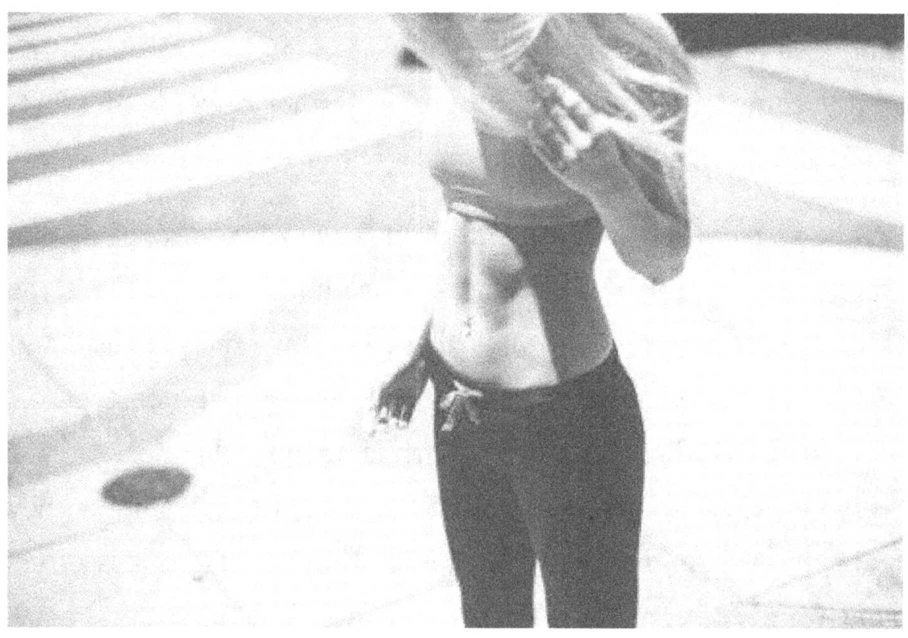

Many people are struggling with weight loss so much that we get frustrated if things do not work out despite our efforts and trials. Medical issues are contributing to the inability to lose weight, genes also play a significant role, and sometimes lifestyle one is exposed to. We blame our environment and other external factors on why we do not lose weight. However, it is important to note that our mind plays a significant role because some of those reasons only exist in our heads. It is not possible to see emotional barriers concerning weighing loss since most of them are not visible. Before we embark on meditation for weight loss, we need to identify and understand those emotional barriers. Also, be very honest with yourself, follow the barriers effect on you, and find out if other psychological factors are also contributing to the same. Understanding these factors helps you be in a better position to tackle them and make better future choices.

While tens of thousands of Americans each year, vow shed some weight, they rarely do because they are not willing to make the sacrifice to do so. They are distracted by other things, and weight loss does not get the priority it deserves. Some even resort to simple diets or eating a particular food, then lose weight very fast. Once they return to their previous lifestyle habits, they gain the weight they had lost. Meditation to weight loss offers long term solution, but it needs dedication, hard work, and resilience. We have an emotional connection with food and eating habits. There are some foods that we connect with a particular scenario, and there is food that reminds us of something. The psychological nature of weight loss will always be misinterpreted. , and thus, most people think just the right diet is enough to make one lose weight. For instance, you can connect vanilla ice-cream with a good feeling. Emotionally you will be longing for that ice-cream, and the urge to take it will be high as your mind tells you once you have it, everything will be okay.

The psychological well-being also plays a great role in weight loss. In the sense that as we struggle to lose weight and all our efforts do not bear fruit, we tend to think that it is impossible. This negative feeling will not be easy to get rid of, especially if it's already on one's mind. So in meditation, we need more than just thinking but understanding why we are doing it. Meditation releases the negative thoughts and energy outside someone's system and keeps them focused and their brain alert. Understanding brings about acceptance and reduces comparison with others as well as appreciating our efforts. This will, in turn, help one not to be bullied or allow other people to look down upon them. For those doing meditation and have the right weight, they will be able to support others on the journey and help them not lose focus and motivate them to continue pressing on and on. We need to acknowledge the big role psychology plays in weight loss and the need for us to connect to our emotions and mind. The more you meditate, the more it becomes part and parcel of you, and you will appreciate the rewards.

People become emotionally attached to food from infancy through adulthood. Children sometimes get rewarded with snacks or treats for healthy behavior; adults can be treated to dinner. There are so many celebrations across the year from Christmas, Halloween, Thanksgiving, birthdays, and Valentine's Day. All these celebrations are food-focused, and as people eat together, they feel good and happy. It has also been proven that an aroma of a special kind of baked cake can create an emotional connection memory that will last throughout someone's lifetime. Some foods are for nourishment, but others we take just for comfort, depending on how they make us feel. Whenever the brain reacts and feels pleasure for a particular food within our reach, most of the time, we will grab it and eat it. During this time, the brain releases a chemical called dopamine, the process feels perfect, and if we equate the feeling with food, then the outcome will be negative.

High body mass index can be linked to emotional problems like anxiety, depression, and stress. Those emotional issues can make one overindulge after a rough day at the office as a reward for a good feeling. Some people use junks as a coping mechanism when they hear bad news. This habit can be only be improved by the use of meditation exercises to deal with one's emotions, stress, or anxiety. As the practices continue and you pay close attention to your breath and allocate more time for thinking.

Chapter 7 - Daily Weight Loss Meditation

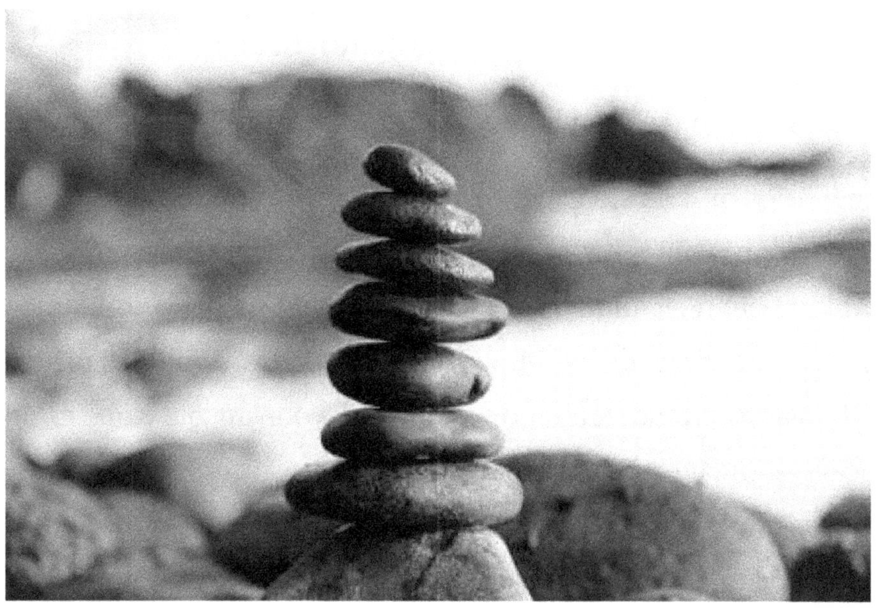

When it comes to rapid weight loss, meditation is one of the techniques that act like secret weapons. Studies conducted on meditation and mindfulness have shown that these exercises are linked to weight loss. They not only boost an individual's awareness but also banish belly fat and lower stress levels. Having an attentive mind can help you avoid binge or emotional eating.

What is Meditation?

Meditation must not be a difficult technique. If you are a beginner, take only five minutes when you wake up to clear your mind before you start off your day. You just need to close your eyes and focus your mind on your goals as you breathe in and out. As you breathe, don't let your mind wander, and if this happens simply guide it back without making any judgment.

What is the Connection between Meditation and Weight Loss?

Meditation is known to be an effective tool for weight loss. It aligns the unconscious mind with the conscious mind in order to facilitate changes that we want to make in our behaviors. Such changes may include avoiding unhealthy foods by altering them with healthier foods. It is important that your unconscious mind becomes engaged in the change process because it is where the weight-gaining, poor habits such as emotional eating are culti-vated. Through meditation, you will be able to become more aware of your surroundings and will be able to overcome your unhealthy habits.

But there is even a more immediate effect of mediation. It can reduce the level of stress hormones in the body. Hormones like cortisol give the body signal to store more calories. If you have high levels of cortisol moving through your system, it is going to be difficult to cut down weight even if you are eating healthy foods. Most of us are stressed in most cases, but it takes only 25 minutes of meditation three times in arrow to reduce the effects of stress.

In 2016, a study that was conducted by Texas Tech University found that increased relaxation, attention, body-mind awareness, calmness, and brain activity result from just a few sessions of meditation. The study also suggested that your self-control could increase with daily meditation. The researchers found that the brain is most affected by meditation, which means that with a few minutes of meditation, you will be able to pass by that ice cream when feeling stressed.

How to Start Meditating for Weight Loss

Even without training, anyone who has a body and mind can practice meditation. For most of us, the most challenging aspect of meditation is getting time. You can start with as little as 8 to 10 minutes a day.

Ensure that you are able to access a quiet place for meditation. If you have children or other people around you, you may need to squeeze time when they are not awake or after they have left the house to avoid distractions. You may even practice your mediation while in the shower.

Once you are in a place of silence, take a comfortable position. You can either lie down or sit in a position that makes you feel at ease.

Start meditating by putting your focus on your breath. Watch the way your stomach or chest rises and falls. Feel the air that you breathe in and out of your mouth. Listen keenly to the sounds around you. This should be done for 2 or 3 minutes until you begin feeling relaxed.

Next, do the following steps:

- Take in a deep breath, and hold for a few seconds

- Slowly breath out, and repeat the process

- Breathe in a natural manner

- Observe the way your breath enters your nostrils, influence the movement of your chest, and moves your stomach.

- Continue focusing on the way you breathe in and out for about 8 to 10 minutes

- Your mind may begin to wonder, which a normal occurrence is. Just acknowledge this and return your attention back to the process

- As you wrap up, reflect on your thoughts, and acknowledge how you can easily bring your mind together

Benefits of Meditation on Weight Loss

Below are the incredible ways that meditation can help you achieve daily weight loss:

1. Meditation reduces stress

With meditation, you will feel calmer as well as have a stress-reducing impact on your body. With endless roles in life including work, children, and home activities, it is not surprising that you may be overwhelmed, which may contribute to increased stress. Unfortunately, these stressors affect your body by producing more cortisol, a stress hormone that affects the levels of sugar and insulin in the body. As a result, the hormone causes weight gain. Studies have revealed that meditation activates a relaxation response, regulating the nervous system and, in turn, lowering the cortisol levels.

With a few minutes of deep breathing and conscious relaxation, you will be able to obtain the cortisol-lowering benefits as well as your overall stress levels.

2. Meditation promotes a focus on intention

Often, meditation techniques involve focusing on specific goals or concepts. Meditating on cutting down weight streams your energy, thoughts, and intentions to a particular goal. In this case, you submit to the intentions by revealing your goals to the world, which makes both your conscious and subconscious mind to be aware of the goal that you want to lose some weight. The outspoken intention will stay with you for a long while, enabling you to achieve your weight loss goal both consciously and subconsciously, and dodging all possible distractions.

3. With meditation, you will learn conscious eating

With daily meditation, you will be able to boost your levels of mindfulness and awareness. This can allow you to live in the moment and always focus on what you are doing in the present. The process of meditation can help you gain an increased sense of awareness of actions and thoughts, thus helping you to think twice before you have taken an action. Rather than enabling your cravings to take over you, you will develop the power of controlling your mind, thus handling your cravings with greater intention and awareness. When you are ready to eat, your awareness will make it easier to recognize the textures and flavors of the food you are eating, instead of taking them for granted.

4. Meditation stabilizes mood hormones

Common daily stressors and activities can affect the way your system operates normally and may throw your hormones out of normal functioning. Apart from keeping your cortisol and adrenaline levels regulated, meditation goes further than this. The technique for relaxation releases both oxytocin and serotonin hormones, which boost your moods and ensure your hormones remain stable.

5. Meditation regulates sleep

Lack of sleep may hinder your weight loss progress. You see, by having a deep sleep, your cortisol levels will rise, which in turn will sabotage your progress in losing weight. Also, when you lack sleep, ghrelin, a hunger signal hormone, is also produced in plenty, thereby increasing your chances of eating more for weight gain. With meditation, you will be able to balance the circadian rhythms that promote quality sleep. Meditation increases the levels of melatonin, a hormone that also determines and controls when you sleep.

How to Make Sure that Meditation Works for You

If you want to include meditation in your rapid weight loss hypnosis, it is important that you make it simple. Meditation should help you recover from any stressful event, not become a source of it. That is why you need to consider the three easy ways highlighted below, which you can incorporate in your daily mediation.

Consider a Mantra That Can Help You Lose Weight

A mantra refers to a phrase that one repeats to focus their mind on mediation and bring them to the relaxation state. A mantra can give help you identify something to focus on as you meditate. Although it is very helpful to many people, a mantra is not a must in meditation. You don't need to force yourself to use one if you don't find it helpful or if it does not make you feel natural. However, in case you choose to use one, you need to repeat it as you inhale as well as when you exhale. Some of the common mantras used include "I am at peace with myself," "I am loved," or "I can do this."

Follow Your Breath to Avoid Stress

As you meditate, try to count your inhales 4 ties and exhales 8 times. Remember that meditation is a process that is aimed at reducing stress; if these counts do not feel natural, you should deviate from them. Every time you meditate, always try to increase the number of exhaling and inhaling counts. Do not feel stressed if it takes longer to reach 8 counts. Just keep in mind that lengthening the exhale will greatly affect your health as you will be able to calm down.

Consider a Guided Meditation

If you are not able to practice meditation alone, you should consider a guided process. This includes websites, phone apps, podcasts, and recordings that can help you connect with experts who guide you on how to meditate.

How to Create a Meditation Space at Home

You may find it easier to practice meditation on a daily basis to motivate your weight loss process. Creating and incorporating meditation accessories and organizing the right space might help you throughout the practice. Some of the equipment to get started including:

Essential Oil Diffuser

Aromatherapy is considered an effective calming tool for the body, which is very helpful during meditation. An essential oil diffuser can help you create a relaxing environment in order to reap the benefits of the essential oils. Additionally, the diffuser always shuts off when the water runs out; thus, you can meditate as long as you like.

Bluetooth Ear bud Headphones

Don't have enough space to practice your meditation? You may consider wireless headphones, which you can to wherever you go. The headphones can sync up with Android and iPhones devices, which you can use to listen to your best-guided mediation without bothering those close to you.

A Meditation Filled Cotton Pillow Cushion

A meditation cushion can give you comfort to find a point of relaxation. The cushion will relieve you from stress, especially after having a prolonged sitting period. It has the perfect density and height to sit through for hours of meditation practice.

Chapter 8 - The Steps on How Hypnosis for Weight Loss Is Done

Hypnotherapists are just like doctors, they have their own way of assessing, evaluating and treating their patients and just like doctors they may also specialize in a particular field. It may be common to have hypnotists that work only for female patients while there are professionals that deal with depression, stress or anxiety – afflicted patients.

This is essential in creating an in depth knowledge on how this important method is done. Only when you are able to understand what happens in an actual hypnosis session will you be able to maximize the true potential of hypnosis.

Inducing relaxation

A hypnotist starts by placing the subject in a room or an area in his office where it is conducive for relaxation or meditation. Hypnosis does not start right away but rather relaxation is achieved first. A hypnotist may ask the person some important questions about himself, some questions regarding his visit and his weight loss. This is important so that the patient is able to establish trust.

As you practice hypnosis, you will need to be in an environment where there is minimal relaxation. You need to focus on what you really need to achieve in your weight loss regimen.

In hypnosis, the patient is not going to:

- Forget anything; he will remember everything that will happen before, during and after the session.

- He is not going to sleep. He will be placed in a very comfortable state but not too comfortable that he would doze off. It is therefore important not to be too tired when practicing hypnosis otherwise you would just sleep during the session.

- He will not be doing anything against his will. Contrary to what was said earlier, hypnosis is not telling someone to jump off a window or to do a chicken dance in front of a crowd but rather it is a personal session between you and a professional and you will not be treated unfairly or made to do something that is against your will.

- He will not lose control and reveal any deep dark secret!

- Finally, he will not be feeling uneasy or weak after the session. There will not just be one but several sessions that will be needed to help a person control his weight gain totally and there will be no side effects whatsoever.

Gaining the trust of the subject does not happen quickly just like gaining trust on a hypnotherapy program. It is normal to have a tinge of skepticism in the treatment while some people may even have second thoughts as to proceed with the procedure. And thus you must explore more on your feelings of fear and anxiety over hypnotism.

With regards to weight loss, the therapist will ask leading questions as to what the subject is feeling towards his weight loss plans and how far he is with his goals. The therapist will find important cues on how to proceed with the therapy such as feelings of depression towards his physical appearance, anxiety over failing, feelings of stress over weight loss, etc. after the therapist has managed to gather enough information about the subject and about his weight loss plans, he will now proceed with the treatment.

On the other hand, you may start with the hypnotherapy session if you are certain with your feelings about your weight loss plans. If you are sure you are ready to proceed with hypnosis, then read on for preparing yourself for the session.

Preparing the subject for hypnosis

The therapist has finally able to gain the subject's trust and confidence and thus proceeds with preparing him for hypnosis. As soon as the subject is ready, he is again placed in a room that is conducive for concentration. This could be a room with minimal lighting, reduced noise and interference from the noisy environment or simply a place where the subject feels calm and relaxed. A therapist may conduct his treatment at his office or in the subject's home or anywhere they may please.

You need to be in a place where there is very little interruption. This will ensure that you will be able to concentrate better and attain relaxation faster too. There are no time frames for preparation. It could take an instant to feel calm while someone that is agitated and stressed could find it hard to keep composed and calm to get ready for hypnosis. Preparation should include the following.

- Making sure that the venue is comfortable. The room temperature should not be too cold or too warm. An uneven room temperature could only distract you.

- You should be lying in bed or sitting on a chair. His hands should not be holding on to anything or holding anything. He should be barefoot and if he is sitting on a chair, the soles of his feet should be touching the carpet or the floor.

- The room should be free from distractions. If the session is to be done at home, you should inform his family that he would be undergoing hypnosis for an hour or more and that he should not be interrupted. Your mobile phone should be powered off or placed on silent mode.

- Playing soft music could be used. Some hypnotists could play music to set the mood while some play rhythmic sounds of nature like running water, wind howling, trickling rain or the sound of waves crashing to the beach.

- The therapist voice helps a lot to set the mood. Most hypnotherapists master the art of talking convincingly as well as softly which helps calm the subject. While practicing the session, whisper or speak in a low tone.

How to induce relaxation

The therapist starts to make the subject, he often feeds some steps to the subject to induce relaxation. You too must practice really well to relax. The success of the hypnosis session depends on how focused you are on the activity and this begins with relaxation.

Here are some basic ways that this is done.

1. Close your eyes and sit still. Your back should be against the back of the chair and your feet should touch the floor. Your hands should be on his lap.

2. You should perform deep breathing exercises. Proper deep breathing exercises start with breathing air deeply through the nose and then holding it for two to three counts. Afterwards, air is expelled slowly

through pursed lips. Repeat this process until you feel relaxed and ready for the next steps.

3. Create a mental image of something or someplace that makes you feel calm. This could be anything like a calm day near the beach or eating hot chicken soup on a rainy day. Recall everything that is to be remembered about that thing for instance, the calm day near the beach would include the gentle sounds of the waves crashing onto the shore, the sound of seagulls nearby, the lingering smell of the sea, the cool morning breeze of the ocean on your face as well as the soft sand on the soles of your feet and in between your toes. Take note of all these in about a few minutes. This mental image will be the triggering point that would help the you take control of your emotions. Every time that you feel uneasy, depressed and out of control, you could recall this mental image to help relax and stay focused.

Now the suggestion is provided

Now that a relaxed state is attained (this is evident through facial expression, body relaxing, hands feeling less tensed and breathing even and deep), the suggestion is now provided. The suggestion is the goal that you want to achieve in your weight loss plan. For instance, you want to lose weight to rekindle your marriage or you want to look great on your wedding day; these solid goals could become instant suggestions that will help guide you towards your goal.

1. Picture yourself finally reaching for your goal. If his goal is to rekindle your failing marriage, you could picture yourself together with your partner and going to places that you two dream of going. The image should be solid just like the mental image that helps you to relax. You must therefore think of your partner warming up to you as well as her appearance, her perfume, her hair, her mannerisms, etc.

2. When you have retained this mental image, you will provide hypnotic suggestions such as "I must stay focused on my goals" or "I must be calm and resist my cravings" or anything that is in line with your goals and aspirations. The suggestion should be repeated as you are in this state of consciousness.

Suggestions vary according to your personal weight loss goals and therefore it is a must to have a clear sense of what you are aiming for or what your ultimate plans are.

Keeping the suggestion in

Now you must keep this hypnotic suggestion in through the help of certain mental images. Remember that there were two images; the first one was an image to relax and the other one was to remind you of your goals. The next image is something or someone that could help keep the suggestion.

One simple way is to think of an object which the subject is familiar with and could remind you of your goals. It could be a pendant, a bracelet or a trinket that you could keep with you wherever you are. To follow our example, you could use a shell pendant on a necklace. Every time you see or touch this pendant you will remember your goals and will tell yourself to keep control over your diet and your exercise regimen. If you wish to slim down for your wedding, you could have your engagement ring as a token to make you remember your goals.

This token should be stated before the hypnosis session is concluded. You need to touch the token just before you open your eyes.

Concluding the hypnotherapy

It is time to awake from your state of heightened awareness and come back to reality. With a therapist, this could be done by telling the subject that upon the count of three, the therapist will snap his fingers two times and the subject should open his eyes.

Reflect on your experience. A single session could last for an hour or more and usually, you will need to repeat the session on more aggressive and more in-depth sessions to help with other aspects of your weight loss plan.

Chapter 9 - The Process of Hypnosis for Weight Loss

Now, you've probably wondered how to do this. You might think it costs a ton of money to go to a therapist to get the hypnosis for weight loss you've wanted. The truth of the matter is, it doesn't take long at all. You can actually do it from the comfort of your own home. It's a great way to allow you to take control of your life, and it's a method that works to allow your body the benefits of hypnosis for weight loss.

Before Entering Hypnotic Trance

You will first need to prepare yourself for the hypnotic trance. You don't want to go into this head-on without any preparation, but you'll want to make sure that you do this right. This is how you get the maximum benefits out of this, and you'll want to do it right.

The first thing to do is to dress for the occasion. You'll want to wear clothing that is comfortable and easy to move in. Don't wear tight things, because that'll just cut off your circulation. It's a quick step to being distracted, and it's something you don't want to deal with. If it's cold, you can wear a loose sweater, but make sure that the hood and hands aren't constricting against your body. Remember, you'll want to be relaxed. Also, make sure you're dressing for the moment. If it's too hot, take off a couple layers. If it's too cold, add a few. Just get your body comfortable.

Next is location. Pick a place where you can just chill and not feel like you're going to be bothered by doing so. You'll feel better when you do that. A good place is the bedroom, or even the living room if you have a comfy couch that is perfect to lay down on. Just make yourself comfortable, and you'll feel better. Occasionally, sitting up works for some because you are more susceptible, but if you're not feeling comfortable, don't do that.

Then, get rid of the distractions. This includes other people. Tell them to go away for a little bit, and you'll be able to relax better. Just tell them that this is your personal time, and they'll understand. Also, turn off all of your electronics. That includes ones in the room you're in. Don't let your hypnotic session become ruined because of a phone call. The less electronics on, the better it'll be. You won't be gone for too long, so it's not the end of the world. '

Another thing to do if people are being distracting is to wear ear buds. You'll be able to have a better time calming down if you take out all sounds from the area. You can then do this without the distractions from life getting in the way.

After that, start looking at your goals. What are you trying to have go away? What are the issues that you have at hand that you need to figure out? You'll want to have these in mind when you're doing this, for they will allow you to have a better time, and it'll allow you to get into the hypnotic state easily.

How to Enter the Hypnotic State

Next is when you enter the state. You have to take various steps to get into there, and this part will tell you exactly what to do. It's important to do this, because failure to do so will not get you anywhere with this technique.

The first thing to do is to close your eyes and just empty your mind. Don't think about the problems you have right now, just get rid of the stress that is laying there. You also want to make sure that you get rid of the feelings of fear and anxiety as well. These will bother you if you don't take care of them, and if you don't handle them adequately, you won't get anywhere. So getting rid of them is your best bet.

To do this, it's best to focus on one thing and think about it. You can clear your head, but it's also best if you just take one thing and think about it, such as how relaxed you are. You can also take one thing in the room and focus on it. After that, you can start to tell yourself that your body is getting heavier. You'll naturally feel this, so just let it continue to go the way it is going.

Now, as you become heady, you'll notice the tension in your body start to form. This is natural, but once you notice it, it'll go away. Do that from the bottom up, and you'll see that your body isn't as heavy as it was before. You'll also notice a release of tension as you do this, and the stress will be less and less as you continue to let your body chill out and go its course.

Once the tension is gone, it's time to breathe. Use meditation breaths, which are slow but deep. This will help you relax better, and you'll be able to let the tension go away. You can visualize the tension leaving the body and going to a better place with breaths, but just make sure they're slow, and through your nose and mouth.

Next is the imagery. By this point, you're fully realized. Now it's time to think of a set of stairs going into a pool of water. Start imagining yourself going down them, and by the time you reach the fifth stair, you'll notice that there is water. Continue to count down from fifteen to one, and soon, you'll feel the tension leave the body, and the relaxation will follow. Keeping relaxed is what will allow you to enter the hypnotic state fully.

Some people recommend tapes and CDs that have meditation and hypnosis techniques, but those are distracting. It's best if you do this on your own, and you'll be able to enter the hypnotic trance easier.

After that, you'll be at the bottom of the water. Step in, and you'll feel like you're floating. You might be spiny as well, but it's a weird sensation that feels good too. You can then start to move into the next part of this, where you imagine a door across the other side. You should visualize yourself wading across it and going through, and at this point, you'll start handling your body and the issues with it.

The Subconscious

Now, you'll imagine your subconscious. This can be whatever you want, but you'll start talking to it. You will want to talk to this entity in a literal manner, but making sure you don't use any negative statements. The first thing that might come to mind is that you need to tell them how you're not going to eat these bad foods, but the problem is, you're going to mess yourself up if you don't do this in a positive fashion. To do this, say positive things to yourself, such as getting a goal weight, or eating a certain amount of calories. It's tricky at first, but if you prepare yourself, you'll be able to get a better result. You can give your subconscious as many statements as you desire, but it is better if you don't overwhelm the apparition with the demands. It's easier on you and your subconscious.

Time to Go!

Now it's time to go. It was fun, but it's time to go back to reality. This is simple, but take it slow. You don't want to go too fast, or it might overwhelm you. Just imagine now that you're back at the door. You're going into the water, and you'll let it submerge you. You'll start to walk up, feeling heavy as you go along. Just keep on going until you're at the top, and soon, the feeling will go away. It'll be an interesting feeling, but it'll make you feel relaxed.

After that, open your eyes. You can tell your body that it's time to get up, or you're going to wake up. You might need to take a little bit to open your eyes, but it'll be fine after a bit. You can imagine that there is a light there as well to help you open your eyes. By doing this, you'll be back in reality and feeling better than ever before.

Hypnosis for weight loss is a great thing to have. It will make it easier on you, and you'll be able to relax the body with this amazing technique. By doing this, you'll be able to relax the body and help change the way you think. It's a great way to kill two birds with one stone, and by the end of it, you'll feel better and have a much better life. Those pounds will shed fast, and you'll be happy that they did.

Chapter 10 - Weight Loss Hypnosis Session

Allowing yourself to relax when thoughts enter your mind you simply choose to acknowledge them then return your attention to the sound of my voice and the sound of my voice goes with you and remains the most important sound you hear.

You are beginning to experience a deeper level of relaxation. I would like you to begin now to focus your attention to your breathing for deeper level of relaxation and the sound of my voice goes with you and every word taking you deeper and deeper, and I really do not know exactly what your own internal state is bringing to you now whether images, sensations or sounds as you listen to each of these words I say to you now with quietness and peace about what you experience now you can practice this experience by believing that you will lose the amount of weight that you want to lose you will lose the correct amount of weight you wish to lose and you are able to do this easily and naturally through mindfully eating healthy and nutritious food.

You feel very proud of yourself you reflect on all the positive things in your life and you know that you will create the most healthy and positive life for yourself and now see yourself clearer on the screen, stomach flat, hips and thighs slim and trim, legs slim and trim, you look great and feel so good you are relaxed and happy, comfortable in your skin and your subconscious mind knows of a time when you only ate to satisfy hunger and you returned now from this moment on to only eat when you are truly hungry.

Your subconscious mind knows exactly how this feels and that this is the best and healthiest way of eating that you will only eat when you are truly physically hungry you only eat when you feel actual physical hunger in your body and when you feel this true hunger you eat healthy vital food that you know is good for your mind good for your body good for your soul and you know when you are truly hungry because it is a hunger that comes on gradually.

True hunger and is easily satisfied with small portions of food and embrace change and growth and maintain awareness of the present moment through emotions and feelings in a deep sense of calmness and peace that enables you to eat slowly while aware of the amount you are eating and chewing and feel satisfied from one meal to the other losing weight steadily safely and naturally when you remain aware of what when and how you eat you are confident in the choices you make about how you look so see yourself now walking outside on a bright fresh day perhaps feeling pride and full of energy for the choices you made to eat healthily you radiate vitality and feel fit and slimmer.

You experience your own feeling in a calm and confident state for your health choices and increase your feeling of health and energy and now it is the moment to end this state in a moment I will count back from one to five and you will come up and out of hypnosis bringing all the benefits feeling yourself coming out slowly now one, one, two, three, four, beginning to move and stretch, and five, eyes open wide away feeling good and anchored in each of folding moment of the present.

With the help of powerful affirmations and visualization, you can achieve your ideal weight in the most natural way.

Avoid concerning yourself with what you eat or not but with how you wish to look.

Do not visualize about disgusting eating or loathing some kind of food.

By saying strong and positive affirmation you make the subconscious mind direct you to eat the right quantities of food with moderation.

Chapter 11 - How to Boost Your Motivation to Work Out

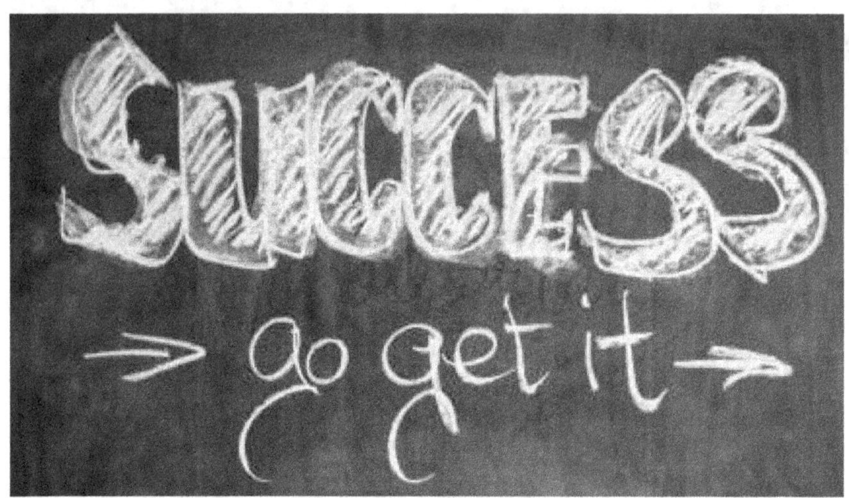

There are two major components of weight loss; your diet and your daily activities. To lose weight, you should eat just enough food to keep you energized for your daily activities.

We will focus on building your motivation to keep exercising. Keeping an active lifestyle will increase your metabolic rate. It will make your body burn more energy even when you are resting.

To be able to integrate workouts to your lifestyle however, you should make sure that you enjoy them. If it feels too much like work, it will be too difficult to maintain. There will come a time

that your mind will be defeated by the distractions and tempta-
tions around you.

Set Realistic Goals and Make a Plan to Reach Them

Before you can start lifting weights, jogging or doing other types of activities, you should put in writing what you want to achieve. If you want to lose weight, you should set the exact number of pounds that you want to lose and the amount of time that you have to achieve your goal. You could also set your goals on specific body parts like your waistline or your arms.

Following the S.M.A.R.T. philosophy to set goals is an ideal tool to use. This ensures goals are Specific, Measurable, Attainable, Realistic and have a Timeline. You should then find a workout plan that fits your schedule and your personality. You should consider the time that you have for your workouts and the effort that you can devote to it.

Remind Yourself of the Benefits of Working Out

Being aware of the benefits of working out will help you continue to do it. You will also be able to build your will power to avoid being lazy. This will remind you that you are not doing this just to look great but also to become healthier.

Make a List of Activities That You Enjoy

If you love dancing, you should include that into your workout plan. If you prefer sports, you should train for the type of sport that you want to participate in. By doing things that you like, you will be able to transition to an active lifestyle with much more ease.

Include a Variety of Activities in Your Workout Plan

Aside from doing what you love, you should also make it habit to try new things and to vary the activities in your workout plan. Lifting weights or running all the time will become boring after some time. If your body is not presented with a challenge every time, it will no longer improve.

Prepare the Necessary Equipment and Outfits

Spending for your workout plan is like investing in your body; you will be expecting a return on your investment. Not only will you feel like an athlete, but this will make you work harder and become more disciplined in following your strategies.

Make Your Workouts a Social Activity

You should avoid doing everything by yourself. Just like in your diet plan, you should also include the people around you. Join people who also like to work out. Motivation, enthusiasm and positive thinking are contagious. You will have a better chance of continuing your weight loss program if you have these people around.

Analyze the Factors That Motivate You

You should also use your metacognitive abilities to improve your performance. Every time you feel extra motivated, you should analyze the internal and external sources of your motivation. Being aware of these factors will give you insights about how your mind works. You can use some of these factors to stimulate your motivation when you are feeling down.

Reward Yourself For Reaching Your Goals

Rewards are things that you allow yourself to have when you reach a certain goal. They are expected to increase the likelihood that you will repeat your positive behaviors. You should decide on the rewards that you will give yourself when making your goals. The thought of the reward will help motivate you. In times when the workout routine becomes hard, you should remind yourself of the reward that you will get if you push through.

You should make sure however, you will be able to follow through with your promise. The most important promises are the ones that you give to yourself.

The only thing that is standing between you and the body you want is mental blocks so, to get over those speed bumps and avoid the inevitable excuses, follow these top methods for rebooting your workout and your mental and emotional state.

You Think – my scales are stuck, why am I bothering?

Rethink - This podge will go

Stick with it. Weight loss is never consistent and the scales, unless they are cheap or faulty, will never lie. First off, the more weight you have to lose, the quicker it will come off – IN THE BEGINNING. After that, it will all start to slow down. Most people reach a weight loss plateau, where they don't lose any weight for several weeks and it is at this point that you must not give in.

One more important point – do not weight yourself every day, it's a very bad habit. Your weight will go up and down daily but it will go down overall. Weigh yourself once a week or fortnight. That way, any loss in weight is a much bigger motivator. Weighing yourself daily is the best way to demotivate yourself so don't do it. Just because you aren't losing any pounds, doesn't mean that your body isn't losing inches and the only way to tell that is how your clothes fit. Give yourself plenty of credit for how much better you look and use that as your motivation to continue.

Redo - Move your routine up a gear

As you lose weight, your metabolism will alter to accommodate the lighter smaller you. That means you are going to have to change the way you encourage your body to burn fat and shed pounds. If you are already on a light diet of around 1500 calories a day, don't cut any more off. Instead, make your workouts more intense and work out for a bit longer each time. Not only will this result in more calories being burned off, it will also make your cardio capacity much larger. This means that you will find it easier to exercise and will be motivated to work out for just that little bit longer. Crank up the resistance on the stationery bike, set the treadmill at more of an incline, walk for a bit longer than you do now, walk at a faster pace or go for one-minute interval runs. Between toning exercises, fit in a set of jumping jacks, running on the spot or step-ups.

You Think - I really can't manage another rep

Rethink - Don't my biceps look fantastic!

If you need a motivational boost, a bit of a lift, psych yourself up mentally and emotionally while you are training. This can increase your muscle power by up to 8% s well as their size and bigger muscles result in an increase in metabolism, which burns off fat faster. So if you needed just one bit of motivation, there it is. Mental imagery is a wonderful boost – when your arms or legs feel tired, imagine bigger and stronger muscles, tell yourself how great you look and you will get another rep or two out.

Redo – Take it down a notch

If you really can manage another rep at the same rate, lighten things off a bit. If you are lifting weights, knock the weights down by 10% until you know you can do another rep in good form. If you are sprinting circuits, slow it down for the last one. The more effort you put in, the better the rewards will be so, even if your final rep is at a lower rate than the older ones, it's still more effort and it will reap rewards. Don't ever beat yourself up if you can't do it but keep this in mind – pushing your limits a little further will get you results you never dreamed of seeing.

You Think - I can't run a mile!

Rethink – That jogger looks like Brad Pitt/Angelina Jolie – whoever takes your fancy at the time really!

When you are slogging your way through that mile, turn your thinking to what is going on around you. Yes, you may slow down a little but you will keep on going and you will finish that mile. Repeat a mental mantra over and over again – something like "I am a running machine" and you will find that you can go for longer and further.

Redo – Divide and Conquer

If you are running a mile, to start with split it up into some bits running and some walking. Jog for maybe quarter of a mile and the walk for a further half mile before jogging the final stretch. As you get better and fitter, as well as leaner, you can jog for further and gradually cut down the walking time. If you can do this three times a week, it won't take long before you can run the entire mile. Your motivation? Your fitness and how you look. Think about how much better you feel and you will keep on going. Do set up a routine for running though. If you only go as and when, it will not work.

You Think - I've damaged my knee/leg/arm etc., I won't be able to do any exercise for a month

Rethink – Where did I put that Pilates DVD?

If you injure yourself and stop working out, it takes a maximum of three days for your body to start losing its conditioning. If that isn't enough motivation of you to get up and go, tell yourself this – there's more than one way to reach that goal. Start by making a list of all the negative thoughts you are having and then turn them into positive thoughts. For example, "I can't go to my exercise class tonight, everything I've done will all go to waste" could be turned into "oh well, now I can start using that Pilates DVD I bought".

Redo – Switch things out

Your regular exercise class might be out but there are other options that are low or no impact. Depending on what injury you have sustained, a bit of moderate training on the elliptical bike can burn off up to 416 calories a hour, water jogging can bur 512 calories an hour as can cycling. These are all good alternatives but only if your injury allows it. If you can't exercise because your legs are injured or you have knee pain, you can still exercise the upper part of your body with hand weights. You can still sit on a chair and punch a boxing bag and Pilates is a form of exercise that is gentle yet effective, designed to allow the maximum benefits in a safe way.

Chapter 12 - Hypnosis for Natural Weight Loss

It can be tempting to give into the promises we see from celebrities and other big brand ads about losing weight. They make it seem so effortless and fun, but when we start the journey ourselves, we soon discover that it is not so simple. This hypnosis is a process that will aide in your weight loss journey and provides for you a natural way to shed the pounds.

You will be guided through the process of feeling better, mindful eating, goal-oriented thoughts, and dedication to the body. This hypnosis is a little different than others and will involve "I" statements. Allow these thoughts to come into your brain as if they were your own.

Natural Weight Loss Hypnosis

Narrator: First you will need to find a calm and quiet place with little distraction. Lay down flat on the ground or bed, or sit with your legs crossed and back comfortably straight, your palms face up and resting on your knees. Once you are in this position begin taking long deep breaths from the stomach, in through the nose, and out the mouth.

Narrator breathes with listener for 5 seconds

Narrator: Good. As you breathe focus in on each of your muscles, letting them constrict and then retract. Move on to the next one. Constrict, retract. Once all of your muscles are relaxed and your mind has focused on your inner and outer breaths, you'll want to clear your mind of all distractions. Imagine as you exhale, all the worries in your life leave with that one outward breath. Continue this until your mind is completely clear and your breath naturally falls into a rhythm.

Narrator pauses for 3-5 seconds

Narrator: As you continue to focus on these breaths, listen to the words carefully, repeat them in your head if you need to. These are affirmations that will change the way your mind thinks about weight loss and a healthier you. I do not need to participate in any diet plan. I do not need to sign up for one specific workout. I am able to go through with the weight loss all on my own. I am capable and ready to lose the weight naturally, using my own body to do this.

Narrator pauses for 3 seconds

Narrator: My body was designed to keep me as healthy as possible. The first step is deciding that I want to lose weight. This is a step that I have already agreed to. I have continually wanted to lose weight and have this be a part of my lifestyle.

Narrator pauses for 3 seconds

Narrator: I am devoted to making the best decision possible for my health. I am learning self-control and focusing on knowing what the best thing for my body is going to be. I understand when I should say "no," and when I need to push myself through something that might be a bit more challenging. I have recognized what bad habits I have done in the past, and I have created new habits that I can start to add to my future.

Narrator pauses for 3 seconds

Narrator: I understand why I need to lose the weight. I am no longer doing this just for looking good. I am doing this because I need to be healthier. I want to feel good all the time. I want to be able to have confidence and love myself easier.

Narrator pauses for 3 seconds

Narrator: I recognize that I need to love myself in this present moment. I cannot do this journey if I do not believe in myself. I am my own trainer. I am the person that is going to be encouraging me more than anyone else. I am the one who is going to be holding all of the power over my life for the rest of my time on this Earth. I am the one who needs to remember the things that are most important for achieving my dreams.

Narrator pauses for 3 seconds

Narrator: I love myself more than I ever have, which is why I am making this journey. If I do not learn to accept myself the way I am right now, then I will never fully be able to love the person that I am, even after I have made the transformation.

I am my own best friend. I have the ability to lose all of the weight that I want because it is part of who I am. It is natural for me to lose the weight the way that my body designed me to do so.

Narrator pauses for 3 seconds

Narrator: I am going to eat less calories than what I am used to eating right now. I am going to exercise more than what I am used to doing right now. I am going to do this so I can burn more calories and lose even more weight. I am dedicated to this lifestyle because I deserve it. I am focused on shedding the pounds because of all the various health benefits that come along with being more in shape.

Narrator pauses for 3 seconds

Narrator: I am going to eat foods that are healthy for me. I will not deprive myself of any nutrition. I will eat in moderation, but I will never starve myself. I will make sure not to overeat, but I will never completely keep food from my body.

I will exercise as often as I can. I will push myself on days that I feel like staying home instead, but I will never push myself to a point that I physically hurt myself. I will know when I need to try a little harder, and I will know when it is OK to lighten up.

Narrator pauses for 3 seconds

Narrator: I will learn all of these things through trusting my body. Not only do I have the natural processes to lose weight already inside of me, but I have what is needed to trust myself through my own intuition. I understand the importance of listening to my gut. I recognize how I can read what I need to do, and know what isn't necessary.

Narrator pauses for 3 seconds

Narrator: I have made mistakes in the past, and there were moments where I didn't judge the situation properly. I will always know how to best listen to my voice as I continue to move forward in this life. I will only grow stronger that voice in the back of my head which tells me what to do. I will listen to my conscious and my subconscious and know how to read both in order to get the truth. I will always be prepared to have to face myself and look deep within my character to get to the root of my issues.

Narrator pauses for 3 seconds

Narrator: I will continue to do this because it is going to help me to lose weight. I will always look for ways to improve the natural methods that I can use to shed the pounds. I am confident in my own abilities to say "no" when it is needed. I won't act on impulse and I will always do my best to control my emotions. The better I can have a handle on my emotions, the easier it will be to know what I need to do to reach my goals and achieve my dreams.

Narrator pauses for 3 seconds

Narrator: I am focused on myself. I am doing this for myself. I am taking care of myself.

Narrator pauses for 3 seconds

Narrator: Each promise that I make to myself is one that brings me closer to my goals. I can feel the air coming in and out of my body. I am focused on relaxing, because reducing my stress will be important in achieving my goals. I am making a dedication to my body.

Narrator pauses for 3 seconds

Narrator: I am going to provide my body with all of the healthy food, water, air, and sun that it can get. I am like a gorgeous plant that needs the attention it deserves to have a vibrant and healthy blossom. I am devoted to myself. I love myself. I love my body. I am going to take care of my body. I am ready for the future. I am not afraid. I am accepting of the bad. I am excited for what is to come.

Narrator pauses for 3 seconds

Narrator: Take in several deeper breaths, just focusing on your body, your promises, and your goals. As you begin to bring yourself into the conscious, slowly open your eyes, press your palms together at your chest, and smile.

Chapter 13 - Meditation That Will Burn Your Fats

Our bodies were designed to burn fat. It is the way that they provide the body with energy when we haven't given it enough through the foods we eat. We require more energy when we workout, so our bodies will burn more fat during these processes.

Though it can sound so simple on paper, it will be rather challenging to always include these things in our lives. This meditation is going to help guide you through the journey of getting the body you want, with a visualization exercise to help you see your goals laid out clearly. Listen to this first when you are in a relaxed position in case you become calm to the point of sleep.

After you know how you react, you might include this when you are doing yoga or another form of light exercise to help keep you grounded and relaxed.

Fat Burn Meditation

Narrator: This is a visualization meditation. I am going to take you on a mindfulness journey through your body. To start, ensure that you are somewhere that you can be fully relaxed. You don't want to have any distractions around, and the only thing that you are going to focus on now is the air that is coming in and out of your body.

Narrator pauses for 3 seconds

Narrator: Let your mind go blank. As thoughts begin to creep in, gently push them out with each exhale. Focus on nothing else other than the air that enters your body, and how it exits.

Narrator pauses for 3 seconds, breathing in and out

Narrator: When we count down from ten, you are going to imagine that you are in the middle of the woods. There is a light trail and you are walking down it.

Breathe in for one, two, and three...

And out for three, two, and one...

You will be in the woods in ten, nine, eight, seven, six, five, four, three, two, and one.

Narrator pauses for 3 seconds

Narrator: You are walking through the woods, noticing everything that surrounds you. There are trees, birds, and even a little stream that you can hear the water running from.

You are feeling incredibly good in this moment, healthy and focused. You haven't eaten in a little bit, but you aren't very hungry just yet. You felt your stomach grumble, but it was just a small signal that you need to eat. Nothing is causing you pain or discomfort. You are focused on right now only, and nothing else.

You are walking up a hill now, a slight incline. You feel the burn start to occur in your legs. As you continue to walk, you begin to realize that your body is starting to burn fat.

You don't have to tell your body to do this. You don't have to take a pill to do this. Your body knows how to do it on its own.

You supply it with healthy food that doesn't add as many calories as you need for energy to your body, meaning that you are burning fat faster.

You put it through workouts in order to burn fat. The combination of both of these is helping you to lose weight.

Narrator pauses for 3 seconds

Narrator: You won't notice in the mirror immediately after burning the fat, but you are feeling it immediately in the way your body functions. Each time your stomach growls, you feel it. Every time you take a step, you feel it. As your body is continuing to get stronger and stronger, and push you closer and closer to the goals that you want, you feel lighter and lighter.

Your body is burning more and more fats. You are becoming more and more relaxed, focusing only on your breathing and the good feeling circulating through your entire body. The only thing that you concern yourself with is shedding the pounds.

Narrator pauses for 3 seconds

Narrator: You are only burning fat. You aren't doing anything to add fat, which means that your body's only option is to use what is already there as an energy source.

You consistently make choices to burn the fat from your body. You are always looking for ways to become lighter and lighter. You feel as your waist is getting slimmer and slimmer.

It feels good to drop the weight. It feels amazing to finally let go of all that has been holding you back.

The more weight that you are burning, the easier it is to lose even more. There is nothing that is going to keep you from getting the things that you want in this life. You are working with your body to get the things that you have been hoping for.

Narrator pauses for 3 seconds

Narrator: You continue to walk through the woods with the realization that you are a part of nature just like all that surrounds you. Your body was made in order to keep you as healthy as possible. Now, it is time to train your brain so that it is optimized for health as well.

Your brain will try to do what it thinks is right for your health. It wants you to eat ice cream, so you feel better right now. It wants you to sit on the couch instead of workout so that you can save your energy. Your body is only thinking of the "now."

You are training your brain to think about the future. You are accepting all that surrounds you, and that you are a part of this nature just as the rest. You are connected to the earth and feel the natural processes flow through your body. You are highly aware of all of the things that you need to do in order to keep your body as healthy as possible.

Narrator pauses for 3 seconds

Narrator: Your body feels better and better the further that you walk. Sometimes you feel a slight strain in your legs, but nothing that is painful. It is simply your body doing its best to burn as much fat as possible. It is your body working hard. It is a good pain, one that makes you feel healthier, stronger.

You have water with you that you take a drink of. This is the fuel that helps to keep your body going. You provide it with everything necessary in order to continually work hard.

Your body will always burn fat. It is designed to use what you already have stored within you. Each time you make a healthy choice, it makes you feel healthier.

Every time you do something good for your body, you are burning fat. You continue to burn fat, always feeling lighter and lighter.

Narrator pauses for 3 seconds

Narrator: You are more relaxed now. Your mind understands what it needs to do to be healthy. You are starting to feel lighter every day.

The forest around you is fading.

As we come to the end of the meditation, remember to focus on your breathing. You will either be able to drift off to sleep or move onto other meditations needed for weight loss mindset.

Chapter 14 - What Makes Your Body Gain Weight: Meditation and Daily Habits

People become emotionally attached to food from infancy through adulthood. Children sometimes get rewarded with snacks or treats for healthy behavior; adults can be treated to dinner. There are so many celebrations across the year from Christmas, Halloween, Thanksgiving, birthdays, and Valentine's Day. All these celebrations are food-focused, and as people eat together, they feel good and happy.

It has also been proven that an aroma of a special kind of baked cake can create an emotional connection memory that will last throughout someone's lifetime. Some foods are for nourishment, but others we take just for comfort, depending on how they make us feel. Whenever the brain reacts and feels pleasure for a particular food within our reach, most of the time, we will grab it and eat it. During this time, the brain releases a chemical called dopamine, the process feels perfect, and if we equate the feeling with food, then the outcome will be negative.

High body mass index (BMI) can be linked to emotional problems like anxiety, depression, and stress. Those emotional issues can make one overindulge after a rough day at the office as a reward for a good feeling. Some people use junks as a coping mechanism when they hear bad news. This habit can be only be improved by the use of meditation exercises to deal with one's emotions, stress, or anxiety. As the practices continue and you pay close attention to your breath and allocate more time for thinking.

We eat to survive, and without food, we will die. Our body needs nutrients to function effectively. Eating because one is hungry is different from eating because there is food or one that wants to eat.

We need to train our system in such a way that we eat to curb hunger just the same way we drink water to quench thirst. While food lovers explore different kinds of food, most of them are keen enough to incorporate healthy eating in their diet.

Mindful Eating

This is a framework used to bring back one's relationship with food and eating experiences. In this technique, your presence is vital, and all the senses are engaged. For instance, how the food smells, the taste of the food, how appetizing it looks, and lastly, your body's reaction to the food.

By this, I mean how that particular food made you feel. Mindful eating always incorporates intuitive eating. It makes the body relax and slow down a little bit as we listen to inner cues of real hunger.

Thus, helping us rectify and reduce emotional binge or emotional eating. Mindful eating can lead to weight loss as long as one makes the right food choices. It is a type of eating that is psychologically controlled, and the food portion measured depending on need. In mind eating, it doesn't matter how much food is there.

What matters is the quantity needed at that particular time. Eating thus becomes a response to hunger other than a leisure activity. People who follow this eating method rarely suffer from obesity. They are physically fit and healthy. During eating also there is no rush regardless of whether one is late or not. The chewing is simultaneous and swallowing.

Intuitive Eating

It is a non-diet approach, mind, and body approach to wellness and health. This approach does not encourage dieting but emphasizes listening to the inner body and hunger cues. By trusting our bodies, intuitive healing renews our relationship with food.

Though it does not encourage dieting, it uses nutritional information to make healthy eating choices and habits. By this habit, we, eat because we need to not because we have to, and dietary values are accepted without bias. In this method we rely more on our intuition. Food is used to satisfy a need. Without the inner cue of hunger, no need for food. For those who want to escape the stress of dieting can appreciate this approach since it is effective and practical. There is no connection between emotions and food in this type of eating.

Emotional or Stress Eating

It happens when people start overeating or under food when they are overwhelmed with mixed emotions rather than eating in response to their inner cues. Strong emotions we experience can sometimes prevent us from listening to our physical feelings and thus preventing us from feeling hungry or full.

In such a scenario, food is used as a mechanism of coping, thus reducing the effect of the intense emotion temporarily. This habit is very addictive, and if not controlled, can lead to obesity, rapid weight gain, overeating, guilt, and shame. Stress-related eating disorder, it cannot handle, can make one vulnerable and not comfortable with their body.

This is where meditation plays a significant role because one will be able to handle their stress situation and, therefore, not use food as a coping mechanism.

Stress eating affects millions of people each year, and although not many will admit it can cause food addiction and unhealthy eating choices. As one eats, they believe eating relieve them of stress and often blame other people for their problems. They do not take responsibility for their actions.

They do not see the need to eat healthy because their mind is preoccupied with so many things.

Dieting

Dieting only changes the food you eat for a while and limit your mindset.

Thus, Meditation will help you tap into your inner feelings and respond to your craving with the ability to control yourself.

Not being in a diet also makes you keep your focus because you will be keen on what you eat and how beneficial it is to your body. Meditation for weight loss changes the perception of the mind, which in turn triggers the inner self to respond to the choices and decisions made. Dieting is restrictive and specific on the meals you are to eat.

It challenges the mind to believe that restriction in terms of food is the only path to weight loss. Meditation, however, is a healthy way of letting the mind be free to choose what is best, learn from mistakes, and be able to focus on becoming better. It is possible to gain weight loss once one stops the diet process. It can offer both long term and short-term weight loss needs. However, the disadvantage is you must know the calories to take per serving.

If you do not know, you may take less, and your body will be deprived of the needed nutrient.

Tackling Barriers to Weight Loss

There are so many barriers to weight loss from personal, to medical, to support system and emotional health. Meditation, if incorporated, will bring fruitful and healthy results. Dedication to overcome the challenges and to be focused on achieving your goals is significant. There are so many distractions, especially before you start tour weight loss routine.

It takes discipline and resilience to manage a healthy loss program. We need to give weight loss the priority it deserves. Also, we need to realize the existence of the said barriers and their contribution toward our goal. The barriers will determine our successes and failures.

Set realistic goals

When you set goals, ensure that they are attainable, specific, and realistic. It is effortless to work on realistic goals and achieve them for better results. If the goals are unrealistic; however, the success rate will be low since on will be discouraged. For instance, when starting with meditation, you can start with as little as five minutes a day and gradually increase it daily until you reach the maximum time like sixty minutes.

The same applies to lose weight during the meditation process. You can start focusing on losing a few pounds each week and gradually increase until you reach your goal. As you set goals, however, realize that it is not your fault if they do not work out as you had planned, do your best and keep your focus.

Always be Accountable

Once you have decided to commit to meditation to weight loss, don't shy away from sharing your plan with your support system and family. It is to ensure that the people you share with also reinforce the commitment and form part of the support system. That way, they will feel part of the program and give support whenever there is a need. You can also use apps for reminders and timings; this way, you have a backup plan whenever you forget.

You can also use motivational bands whenever you achieve a milestone set. Being accountable makes you enjoy your successes, acknowledge your failure, and appreciate your support system.

People thrive when they feel responsible for something, especially on something beneficial to their well-being.

Modify Your Mindset

Your thinking needs to be modified in the sense that you be keen on the information you are telling yourself. Ensure that your mind is not filled with unproductive and negative thoughts, which will bring you down or discourage you. Do not be scared of challenging your thoughts and appreciate your body image.

Your mindset determines your thinking and in turn, creates a sense of appreciation or rejection. Our weight loss largely depends on our mindset; do you believe you can do it? If you think you have all it takes, then absolutely nothing will prevent or stop you.

Manage Stress Regularly

Having a stress management technique should be part of one's daily routine. You need to develop a healthy stress-relieving mechanism that can help you live a stress-free life. Understand that meditation is a stress reliever in its own right as it helps calm the mind and soothes the body.

It can be used to manage stress and its benefits fully utilized to live a more productive life. Be able to handle stress efficiently. Stress is not healthy for the mind.

If not handle, it can cause emotional problems and makes one irrational, moody, or violent. Be your own boss when managing your stress.

Be Educated About Weight Loss

As you embark on meditation for weight loss, be educated about how it works; that way, weight loss will not be a struggle.

You will be able to handle failed attempts as well as appreciate the progress made.

You will be able to know what you have been doing wrong and decide on the best meditation exercise for you.

 If you have misleading information, then your general progress may be inhibited

Weight loss need not be too expensive; neither does it require a costly gym membership or enrolment in a costly meditation class. There are various self-practice meditation exercises that you can comfortably do at home. There are various meal plans and diets that may work for others though they may not offer long term solutions or lasting behavior changes. Have the right information that you need. Don't be misled by anyone posing that they are professionals in that field. Also, do not hesitate to do research online and compare notes. From there, you will be able to come back with something that works for you.

Chapter 15 - Your Meditation for a Mindfulness Diet

One of the best ways to transition into a diet that's centered on weight loss is to do so using mindful eating. All too often, we eat well beyond what is needed, and this may lead to unwanted weight gain down the line.

Mindful eating is important because it will help you appreciate food more. Rather than eating large portions just to feel full, you will work on savoring every bite.

This will be helpful for those people who want to fast but need to do something to increase their willpower when they are elongating the periods in between their mealtimes. It will also be very helpful for the individuals who struggle with binge eating.

Portion control alone can be enough for some people to see the physical results of their weight-loss plan. Do your best to incorporate mindful eating practices in your daily life so that you can control how much you are eating.

This meditation is going to be specific for eating an apple. You can practice mindful eating without meditation by sharing meals with others or sitting alone with nothing but a nice view out the window. This meditation will still guide you so that you understand the kinds of thoughts that will be helpful while staying mindful during your meals.

Mindful Eating Meditation

You are now sitting down, completely relaxed. Find a comfortable spot where you can keep your feet on the ground and put as little strain throughout your body as possible. You are focused on breathing in as deeply as you can.

Close your eyes as we take you through this meditation. If you want to actually eat an apple as we go through this that is great. Alternatively it can simply be an exercise that you can use to envision yourself eating an apple.

Let's start with a breathing exercise. Take your hand and make a fist. Point out your thumb and your pink. Now, place your right pinky on your left nostril. Breathe in through your right nostril.

Now, take your thumb and place it on your right nostril. Release your pink and breathe out through your nostrils. This is a great breathing exercise that will help to keep you focused.

While you continue to do this, breathe in for one, two, three, four, and five. Breathe out for six, seven, eight, nine, and 10. Breathe in for one, two, three, four, and five. Breathe out for six, seven, eight, nine, and 10.

You can place your hand back down but ensure that you are keeping up with this breathing pattern to regulate the air inside your body. It will allow you to remain focused and centered now.

Close your eyes and let yourself to become more relaxed. Breathe in and then out.

In front of you, there is an apple and a glass of water. The apple has been perfectly sliced already because you want to be able to eat the fruit with ease. You do not need to cut it every time, but it is nice to change up the form and texture of the apple before eating it.

Breathe in for one, two, three, four, and five. Breathe out for six, seven, eight, nine, and 10.

Now, you reach for the water and take a sip. You do not chug the water as it makes it hard for your body to process the liquid easily. You are sipping the water, taking in everything about it. You are made up of water, so you need to replenish yourself with nature's nectar constantly.

You are still focused on breathing and becoming more relaxed. Then, you reach for a slice of apple and slowly place it in your mouth. You let it sit there for a moment and then you take a bite.

It crunches between your teeth, the texture satisfying your craving. It is amazing that this apple came from nature. It always surprises you how delicious and sweet something that comes straight from the earth can be.

You chew the apple slowly, breaking it down as much as you can. You know how important it is for your food to be broken down as much as possible so that you can digest it. This will help your body absorb as many vitamins and minerals as possible.

This bit is making you feel healthy. Each time you take another bite, it fills you more and more with the good things that your body needs. Each time you take a bite, you are making a decision in favor of your health. Each time you swallow a piece of the apple, you are becoming more centered on feeling and looking even better.

You are taking a break from eating now. You do not need to eat this apple fast. You know that it is more important to take your time.

Look down at the apple now. It has an attractive skin on the outside. You wouldn't think by looking at it about what this sweet fruit might look like inside. Its skin was built to protect it. Its skin keeps everything good inside.

The inside is white, fresh, and very juicy. Think of all this apple could have been used for. Sauce, juice, and pie. There are so many options when it comes to what this apple may have become. Instead, it is going directly into your body. It is going to provide you with the delicious fruit that can give you nourishment.

You reach for your glass of water and take a long drink. It is still okay to take big drinks. However, you are focused now on going back to small sips. You take a drink and allow the water to move through your mouth. You use this water not just to fill your body but to clean it. Water washes over you, and you can use it in your mouth to wash things out as well.

You swallow your water and feel it as it begins to travel through your body. You place the water down now and reach for another apple slice.

You take a bite, feeling the apple crunch between your teeth once again. You feel this apple slice travel from your mouth throughout the rest of your body. Your body is going to work to break down every part of the apple and use it for nourishment. Your body knows how to take the good things that you are feeding it and use that for something good. Your body is smart. Your body is strong. Your body understands what needs to be done to become as healthy as possible.

You are eating until you are full. You do not need to eat any more than what is necessary to keep your body healthy. You are only eating things that are good for it.

You continue to drink water. You feel how it awakens you. You are like a plant that starts to sag once you don't have enough water. You are energized, hydrated, and filled with everything needed to live a happy and healthy life.

You are still focused on your breathing. We will now end the meditation, and you can move onto either finishing the apple or doing something relaxing.

You are centered on your health. You are keeping track of your breathing. You feel the air come into your body. You also feel it as it leaves. When we reach zero, you will be out of the meditation.

Twenty, 19, 18, 17, 16, 15, 14, 13, 12, 11, 10, nine, eight, seven, six, five, four, three, two, one.

Chapter 16 - Work Out Meditation Hypnosis

Sit back comfortably in your chair and take a deep breath in and as you breathe out just close your eyes. Allow your breathing to be normal and natural as you begin to relax right now. Imagine yourself you a moment just feeling completely relaxed. What is it like inside your mind as you go into this relaxing trance?

Just pretend for a moment that you are drifting into a relaxing state of hypnosis and make believe that you are a great subject for hypnosis. What's it like when you are in hypnosis, what is it like when you are relaxing even more deeply now?

Allow that relaxation to spread throughout your body. Allow the muscles around your eyes to relax, allow your jaw to relax. Allow the relaxation to continue to your shoulders, arms, chest and abdomen. Just relax. Allow your spine to relax, your hips, your upper legs, knees, lower legs and feet to just relax completely. Feeling comfortable and relaxed in every way, that's right.

Feel the chair and know that you are completely safe. You may, from time to time hear noises around you and that's ok, it means that you can just relax. Know that wherever you go, my voice will go with you and the meaning of my words will always be clear to you.

And what would it be like if you allow your mind to relax also and your body continues to relax comfortably. Notice that it is as if your mind is taking you on a journey inside. And why not just suppose that this session of hypnosis begins to deepen more and more. Notice that you are experiencing your thoughts changing as if you were floating on the breeze.

I need to tell you that going into hypnosis is the most resourceful experience. So you must take your time to relax your body and your mind fully straight away or in a moment. You should begin by noticing your breathing, your body can relax too and you really should relax completely.

I know you are wondering why you are so relaxed now and you are wondering why your breathing has changed and perhaps your even wondering why your trance has deepen as you are breathing naturally, takes you deeper still. Allow yourself to do that now, so that your inner mind can take you on a journey inside your inner world so that you find yourself going deeper and deeper into hypnosis.

Realize that your body relaxes automatically in all kinds of fascinating ways and realize that this trance is particularly resourceful for you. You can breathe in and out comfortably and your unconscious mind can absorb all kinds of valuable suggestions and pieces of information. That's right.

As soon as you notice your breathing, you'll realize that you are so completely relaxed that your body has been breathing for you all along; as soon as you make that realization you will begin to go even deeper into a very comfortable trance like state.

And your conscious mind to wonder about trance and wonder about this session of hypnosis while it does your unconscious mind can be constructing patterns and integrating learnings while you consciously feel completely and totally relaxed you are unconscious.

Every time you want be clear and concise about your fitness objectives, know that you can achieve your goals successfully because you can align your positive thoughts and energy that will support you in what you want to achieve. Because it is part of you and you find it easy to work out consistently. Feeling totally in control of your thoughts and in control of achieving your fitness objectives through consistent, regular exercise because it comes naturally to you and that means that you can be clear about what you want and achieve what you want. Which means you are motivated and positive and you can achieve all that you want knowing the positive feelings are yours having now experienced that motivation to work out consistently. That means you can access all of the motivation that is yours by right and every time that you do this you are empowered knowing the control that you have over your life and the motivation to work out regularly and consistently puts you in charge allowing you to create the results that you want and to complete your work out goals easily and effortlessly successfully.

 Simply by realizing that you can achieve your work out objectives for yourself means that it's an experience that is familiar to you allowing you to know that every time you want to feel motivated to achieve to your results, you know that the focus and motivation to work out consistently is there because it is part of you and feeling positive, it comes naturally to you and that means that you can comfortably do all that you want knowing that you can work out consistently and move towards your exercise goals. Having now experienced that you have successfully achieved your workout objectives that means you can access all of the resources and learnings that are yours by right and every time that you do this you find it easy to work out consistently and regularly knowing the motivation and positivity is easy to access because it's a resource that you can use easily and effortlessly. It's natural for you and your focus gives you confidence in that.

Because you are in this session of hypnosis that means that the next time you choose to go into hypnosis you will access deeper levels of trance. You are a wonderful person with such a warm and charismatic personality creating such a positive effect on all those people around you as you are realizing now the changes that this journey has created for you.

 I want you to know that you are an incredibly capable and confident individual and that you will achieve all that you want. You have done a good job in making this a valuable and resourceful experience and your unconscious mind has accepted all of the positive suggestions I have given you and you can implement them into your behavior at your own pace.

Chapter 17 - How to Forgive Your Self from Dietary Mistakes

Forgiveness is an underrated and extremely important element of weight loss. Often times, people who are in the position of wanting or needing to lose weight fail to acknowledge the fact that they have been feeling incredibly frustrated with them. Anger, frustration, disappointment, and sadness directed at yourself when you are on this journey are all incredibly normal feelings to have. They can also be painful and overwhelming if you do not take the time to acknowledge them, forgive yourself, and heal them as you experience them.

You may find yourself feeling angry, frustrated, disappointed, or sad that you let yourself gain so much weight. You may fail to acknowledge the fact that it was not intentional, or that it had causes that were beyond your control, especially if your weight gain was related to medical conditions or a lack of education around healthy eating. Regardless of what lead to you gaining weight, you may feel contempt for yourself for "allowing" it to happen, and that may make it difficult for you to commit to losing weight truly. When you sit in anger and frustration with yourself, it can be difficult to accept yourself as you are now and work toward improving your wellbeing through weight loss. Forgiving yourself for not knowing better or for not doing better, or even forgiving yourself for blaming yourself for something that was beyond your control, is important. The more you can forgive yourself, the more likely you are to acknowledge that your weight is something you want to work on. Through that, you will be able to work on weight loss from a peaceful frame of mind.

Studies have shown that those who accept themselves as they are and forgive their mistakes are more likely to lose the excess weight and keep it off than those who refuse to forgive themselves. Refusing to forgive yourself can create a massive amount of stress inside of you that makes it difficult for you to stay focused on exercising, eating healthy, and improving your wellness. Many people find that this difficulty in forgiving themselves worsens their self-esteem and self-confidence, which keeps them in the unhealthy cycle of behaviors and patterns that lead to their weight gain in the first place. If you want to overcome these cycles, you need to be willing to forgive yourself for your past choices, mistakes, and experiences that may or may not have been beyond your control.

Another area where you need to master forgiveness is in the process of change. As you move away from old habits and behaviors and into a new way of looking after your body, you are all but guaranteed to make mistakes. You are going to have days or even weeks where you fall back into old patterns. Some people even fall back into old patterns and stay trapped in them for years. This happens because they are unwilling to forgive themselves for making a mistake, and so they fall back into the cycle of contempt and low self-esteem and self-worth.

If you want to be able to continue moving forward with your wellness and to jump back on track as quickly as possible, you need to be willing to forgive yourself for any mistakes you make. This means anytime you overeat, engage in an old eating pattern, opt for an unhealthy food choice, or otherwise make a "mistake" in your diet, you forgive yourself. Upon forgiving yourself, make sure that you also commit to taking that experience into account so that you can make better choices. Make an honest effort to do better next time so that each time you forgive yourself, you give yourself a reason to believe that your commitment to yourself genuinely means something. When you can forgive yourself and believe that your commitment to bettering yourself and your life means something, you begin to build your self-esteem. Through that, things like portion control begin to become easier, and you find yourself naturally gravitating toward taking better care of yourself.

Chapter 18 - 100 Affirmations to Weight Loss

Weight Loss Affirmations

These are all phrases that you should say to yourself as often as possible. As we read them, let them flow through your mind as if they are your own.

Write the words down to remember those further, put notes around your house with the affirmations written on them, or simply find other creative ways to incorporate these affirmations in your life. Let's start reading them now so that you can get these ideas in your head right away.

Positive Affirmations for Weight Loss

1. I am healthy, wealthy and clever

2. I let go of the illness, i am not ill

3. Thanks to my creator and everyone in my life.

4. I am grateful for all the bounty that I already enjoy

5. Every day I grow energetically and vibrantly

6. I only give my body the necessary nutritious food

7. My body is my temple

8. You can always maintain a healthy weight

9. I deserve to enjoy perfect health

10. Act to be healthy

11. I respect my body and am willing to exercise

12. Affirmation For Rapid And Natural Weight Loss

13. My body is beautiful and healthy

14. I choose healthy and nutritious foods

15. I like to exercise and I do it frequently

16. Losing weight is easy and even fun

17. I have confidence in myself

18. I am now sure of myself

19. I feel confident to succeed

20. From day to day, I am more and more confident

21. I am sure to reach my goal

22. I want to be a noble example

23. I believe in my value

24. I have the strength to realize my dreams

25. I am really adorable

26. I trust my inner wisdom

27. Everything I do satisfies me deeply

28. I trust the process of life

29. I can free the past and forgive

30. No thought of the past limits me

31. I get ready to change and grow

32. I am safe in the Universe and life loves me and supports me

33. With joy I observe how life supports me abundantly and provides me with more goods than I can imagine.

34. Freedom is my divine right

35. I accept myself and create peace in my mind and my heart

36. I am a loved person and I am safe.

37. Divine Intelligence continually guides me in achieving my goals

38. I feel happy to live

39. I create peace in my mind, and my body reflects it with perfect health

40. All my experiences are opportunities to learn and grow

41.   I flow with life easily and effortlessly

42. My ability to create the good in my life is unlimited

43. I deserve to be loved because I exist

44. I am a being worthy of love

45. I dare to try and I'm proud of it

46. I choose to really love myself

47. I love myself and accept myself completely

48. I am ready to try new things

49. There are things I can already do, I just need to start even though I'm not ready yet

50. I am much more capable than I think

51. As I love myself, I allow others to love me too ...

52. I accumulate more and more confidence in myself

53. I am unique and perfect as I am

54. I am wonderful

55. I'm proud of everything I've accomplished

56. I do not have to be perfect, I just need to be myself

57. I feel able to succeed

58. I give myself permission to go out of my role as a victim
and take more responsibility for my life

59. The past is over, I now have control of my life and I move

60. I am my best friend

61. I am able to say "no" without fear of displeasing

62. I choose to clean myself of my fears and my doubts

63. Fear is a simple emotion that cannot stop me from suc-
ceeding

64. Every step forward I make increases my strength

65. My hesitations give way to victory

66. I want to do it, I can do it

67. I am capable of great things

68. There is no one more important than me

69. I may be wrong but that I can handle it

70. With confidence, I can accomplish everything

71. I allow myself to have a lot of fun

72. I deserve to be seen, heard and shine

73. I deserve love and respect

74. I choose to believe in myself

75. I allow myself to feel good about myself and trust myself

76. I reduce measures quickly and easily

77. I can maintain my ideal weight without many problems

78. My body feels light and in perfect health

79. I'm motivated to lose weight and stay

80. Every day I reduce measures and lose weight

81. I fulfill my weight loss goals

82. I lose weight every day, and I recover my perfect figure

83. I eat like a thin person

84. I treat my body with love and give it healthy food

85. I choose to feel good inside and out

86. I feed myself only until I am satisfied, I don't saturate my food body

87. I know how to choose my food in a balanced way.

88. I feed slowly and enjoy every bite.

89. I am the only one who can choose how I eat and how I want to see myself.

90. It is easy for me to control the amounts of what I eat.

91. I learn to have habits that lead me to my ideal weight.

92. Being at my ideal weight makes me feel healthy and young.

93. My body is very grateful and quickly reflects all the care I have with him.

94. My body reflects my perfect health.

95. I feel better every day

96. Being at my ideal weight motivates me to do other things that I like.

97. The human body is moldable, and I am the (the) artist of my body.

98. Every day I eat with awareness.

99. I consume the calories needed to have an ideal weight and a healthy body.

100. Every day I like the way I feel.

Chapter 19 - How to Use Affirmations, Meditation and Hypnosis for Weight Loss Naturally

How Do I Pick and Use Affirmations for Weight Loss?

Choosing affirmations for your weight loss journey requires you first to understand what it is that you are looking for, and what types of positive thoughts are going to help you get there. You can start by identifying what your dream is, what you want your ideal body to look and feel like, and how you want to feel as you achieve your dream of losing weight. Once you have identified what your dream is, you need to identify what current beliefs you have around the dream that you are aspiring to achieve. For example, if you want to lose 25 pounds so that you can have a healthier weight, but you believe that it will be incredibly hard to lose that weight, then you know that your current beliefs are that losing weight is hard. You need to identify every single belief surrounding your weight loss goals and recognize which ones are negative or are limiting and preventing you from achieving your goal of losing weight.

After you have identified which of your beliefs are negative and unhelpful, you can choose affirmations that are going to help you change your beliefs. Typically, you want to choose an affir-mation that is going to help you completely change that belief in the opposite direction. For example, if you think "losing weight is hard," your new affirmation could be "I lose the weight effort-lessly." Even if you do not believe this new affirmation right now, the goal is to repeat it to yourself enough that it becomes a part of your identity and, inevitably, your reality. This way, you are anchoring in your hypnosis sessions, and you are effectively rewiring your brain in between sessions, too.

As you use affirmations to help you achieve weight loss, I en-courage you to do so in a way that is intuitive to your experience. There is no right or wrong way to approach affirmations, as long as you are using them on a regular basis. Once you feel yourself effortlessly believing in an affirmation, you can start incorporat-ing new affirmations into your routine so that you can continue to use your affirmations to improve your wellbeing overall. Ide-ally, you should always be using positive affirmations even after you have seen the changes you desire, as affirmations are a wonderful way to help naturally maintain your mental, emo-tional, and physical wellbeing.

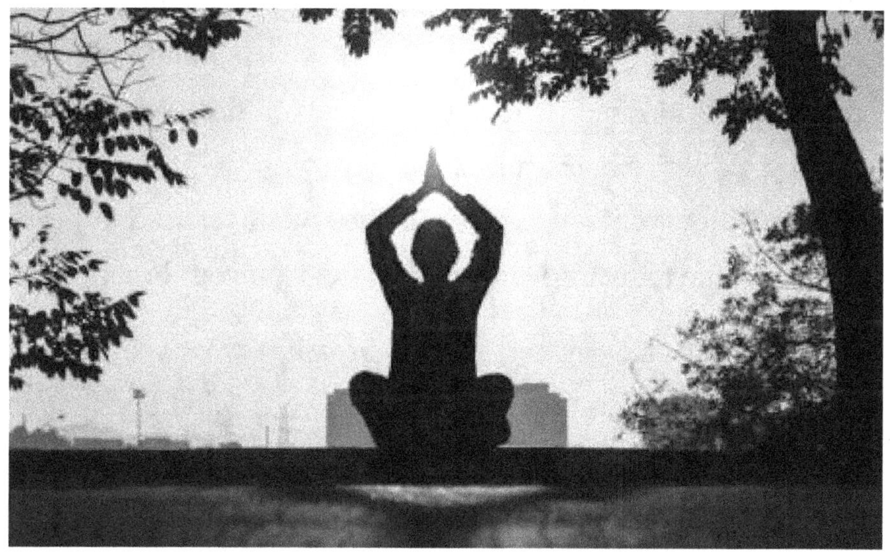

To begin this meditation, I want you to start by sitting or lying down in a comfortable place where you can breathe in and out freely. As you do, focus on your breath, and allow yourself to begin to become one with this present moment. Feel yourself sinking into the present with each breath as you anchor yourself into the here and now. Breathe in, feeling yourself connecting with your body, and breathe out, feeling yourself connecting with this moment. Allow yourself to enjoy the space and freedom of this moment as you indulge in the betterment of yourself and your mind.

As you begin to feel yourself relaxing, I want you to focus even deeper now on your breath. Each time you feel your thoughts being drawn away to something else, gently, and lovingly bring them back to your breath. Feel your chest rising and falling as you breathe in and out. Notice how it feels to have each breath nourish your entire body, mind, and soul with the loving energy of oxygen. Allow yourself to be supported by this natural process as you continue to focus deeply and lovingly on your breath.

While you continue to focus on your breath, I want you to keep an open mind for what is to follow. Feel your mind opening as you breathe in, allowing space for new thoughts that will nurture and support you. Allow any negative or unwanted thoughts to disappear with each exhale naturally. Continue this pattern, now.

In your open mind, repeat after me, while continuing to follow your breathing pattern:

"I am in control.

I have the power to decide.

I am in control of my desires.

Self-control comes easily to me.

I can tap into self-control whenever I need to.

I see things through to the end.

I love moving my body.

Today, I will have an excellent workout.

I have a strong body and mind.

My body is becoming healthier every single day.

I am transforming my body every day.

I am losing weight daily.

I am dedicated to taking care of my body.

I choose to eat only healthy foods.

I rest when my body needs rest.

I love leading a healthy lifestyle.

I am always doing the best I can.

I make healthy choices.

I love myself.

I praise myself freely.

I appreciate myself.

I love my body.

I am willing to change to become the best version of myself.

I am a beautiful person.

I treat my body with the respect it deserves.

I am uniquely beautiful.

My beauty is innate.

My entire self is beautiful.

My beauty shines for all to see.

I am naturally beautiful."

As you continue breathing, allow these words to percolate in your mind. Feel them becoming one with who you are, with your identity. Feel yourself affirming that you are, indeed, a strong, capable, beautiful, worthy, and fit human being that can effortlessly lose the weight that you desire to lose. Feel yourself lovingly accepting this new, healthier version of yourself. Allow yourself to become one with this new image of you. Believe the words and affirmations that you have repeated back to yourself and trust that they are true. Commit to believing them.

When you are ready, you can begin to bring your awareness back into the room around you. Allow yourself to open your eyes, return to a natural breathing rhythm, and prepare for the day ahead of you. As you do, feel yourself believing in every single affirmation you heard today, and trusting that it is completely, absolutely true.

There is an amazing measure of logical research that takes a gander at the viability of weight reduction mesmerizing, and a lot of it is sure. One of the underlying 1986 research found that overweight females utilizing a mesmerizing project shed 17 pounds contrasted with 0.5 pounds for females just advised to watch what they ate. A mesmerizing weight reduction study meta-investigation during the 1990s found that members who utilized trance lost more than twice as much weight as the individuals who didn't. Also, an examination in 2014 found that females who utilized entrancing were improving their weight, BMI, eating conduct, and even certain parts of self-perception.

In any case, it's not all uplifting news: A Stanford study in 2012 found that about a fourth of individuals just can't be mesmerized, and it has nothing to do with their characters, as opposed to basic conviction. Or maybe, the minds of certain individuals simply don't appear to work that way. "In case you're not inclined to staring off into space, you regularly think that it's difficult to stall out in a book or endure a motion picture, and don't believe you're innovative, you may be one of the individuals for whom trance isn't functioning admirably," says Dr. Stein.

Georgia is one of the examples of overcoming adversity. She guarantees it helped her lose the extra pounds as well as helped

her keep them off also. After six years, she kept her weight reduction joyfully, now and then returning in with her trance spe-
cialist when she requires a boost.

Conclusion

Thank you for making it to the end. Do you remember the shocking first time when you couldn't button your favorite jeans effortlessly? Do you run out of steam while having fun with the kids? Do you lack fitness for a carefree bike tour through the green? Do you avoid such situations because you simply carry too much weight with yourself and no longer feel comfortable in your skin?

There are many reasons for wanting to lose excess kilos. Numerous diets promise you maximum success with minimal effort. Such radical cures are mostly very one-sided, associated with deficiency symptoms, and only effective for a short time. If the yo-yo effect comes, your body size quickly increases again, but your well-being decreases.

Under hypnosis, you're eating habits, thinking patterns, and behaviors are checked and permanently changed. Without sacrificing enjoyment, sweets and fats are becoming increasingly unattractive for you. Instead, you feel more motivated and want to exercise and eat healthy food. Instead of the chocolate bar, you'd better grab the bike. With every dwindling kilo, you gain satisfaction, health, and quality of life. The pounds drop, and you feel relieved.

Some people eat for emotional reasons to compensate for boredom, loneliness, or grief. Others suffer from a lack of exercise, associated with an excess of calories and low metabolism. Some people just eat unhealthily. Often, due to lack of time, they resort to industrially manufactured food that, in addition to very high fat, sugar, and salt content, primarily supplies empty calories. It's quick to snack here and eat there on the side.

The focus is on work or the television program - the perception of one's body signals such as hunger or satiety fades into the background and is forgotten. Stress is also one of the major factors that must be considered when fighting obesity.

Many causes of obesity are on a mental level, where behavioral patterns, ways of thinking, motivation, and discipline are anchored. It is difficult to break through this spiritual level or to control it via the rational mind. And this is exactly where hypnosis for weight loss comes in.

Under hypnosis, you are in a trance-like, changed state of consciousness.

Meanwhile, your subconscious mind is more responsive and more receptive to positive messages. Hypnosis takes advantage of this condition - to influence the difficult to access mental areas and reconfigure them for your benefit.

Thanks to the way it works, hypnosis helps you achieve your individual goal. If you are an emotional eater, it can be used, for example, for deep hypnotic relaxation to reduce stress and to change your eating habits. In future stress and frustration situations, unhealthy foods will then be of no interest to you, and your diet will level out healthily. The hypnotist gains new motivation and desire for calorie-burning activities. Whatever your obesity may be: hypnosis for weight loss, you approach your weight loss goal step by step. Without having to forego eating pleasure, you develop new body awareness, zest for life, satisfaction, and joy in losing weight.

DEEP SLEEP

A COMPLETE GUIDE TO POWERFUL GUIDED MEDITATION AND DEEP SLEEP HYPNOSIS WITH PRACTICAL EXERCISE TO REDUCE STRESS AND ANXIETY

Emily Anderson

Emily Anderson

Introduction

We humans mostly live in our mind, on automatic pilot mode. Where we do not control our thoughts, letting them jump from one to the next one. We do not live in the present most of our time. Our thoughts are like cars on the road. There are plenty of them. And we cannot stop or control them. But When we try to control them. Our mind gets busy by the overwhelming pressure of it, and it increases the feeling of restlessness. And therefore, we need meditation: to tame our mind. Meditation is a skill to teach our mind how to be less distracted. It teaches our mind how to relax, how to do nothing, and most importantly, how to enjoy the moments of stillness with all the thoughts behind.

How to Meditate?

Meditation is way easier than people think because the only hard thing is to take some time out. Once you do this, the next steps are already easy for you. Although there are many types of meditation, this one particularly is breathing exercise. In this meditation, the only focus will be on the breath, how our body inhales and exhales the air. This two-to-five-minute activity has long-term benefits. It improves our attention span, promotes calmness, and many more. One can repeat it as many times as he wants to help himself get rid of distractions and increase focus.

By starting, go through these steps one by one. It probably seems hard for the beginner, but try to complete the steps by doing your best.

So, what you have to do is to get a few minutes out and follow these steps.

- The First thing you have to do is to leave everything aside, switch your phone off and find a place where you will not get distracted easily. Sit on the floor in a comfortable position.

- Now start noticing your breath. Don't push yourself to breathe deep. Just let yourself inhale in the usual manner and focus your attention on breathing to free your mind from distractions. To do so, gradually close your eyes and notice the sounds of your surroundings.

- By taking a normal breath then take a deep breath. Slowly inhale through your nose until you feel the rise of your stomach and chest. As you breathe in, try to hold it for a few seconds. Breathe out slowly through your mouth. Make sure you exhale longer than inhale. Doing it, when thoughts enter your mind, gently acknowledge them and let them go, and bring your focus on breathing.

- Repeat it two or three times. And by doing it regularly, you will see a change in yourself. You will feel lighter and fresher. Your behavior will also get positive and cooperative. Your mind will be clearer and calmer. You lower your stress level, you control your anxiety, your sleep gets better, and you get familiar with ease and peace of mind. You are getting ever-lasting benefits from doing this.

Chapter 1 - Mindfulness Meditation

But first what is the thing called mindfulness? Mindfulness is a state of mind that makes us live in the present without dwelling in the past or exploring the future. In this state, we control our attention, awareness, and thoughts.it is like "paying attention purposely".it is a non-judgmental approach to observe our thoughts, emotions, and bodily sensations. Two things are required for mindfulness: presence and consciousness. Presence is being "in the now" and consciousness is being aware of the surroundings. We often experience being in a state where we get preoccupied with any of our thoughts and we cannot stop thinking about it. Preoccupation mainly occurs when we are stressed, we are having anxiety and depression. Occupied mind also affects the performance of our body's functions. Mindfulness keeps us in the present, brings us back to the here and now. Mindfulness can be learned through meditation. Mindful meditation is the training of the mind that teaches us to pause the thoughts and calm our mind and body. Science links good mental and physical health with mindfulness.

What is it like to be mindful? Being mindful is being in our senses. It means having attention to any of the five senses. It can be seeing objects, hearing voices, feeling any sensation, or tasting or smelling the food. Be mindful is to be in being mode. Where we are fully aware of ourselves.

There are many mindful meditations. But mainly, all types of meditations involve two things: breathing and consciousness of body and mind. To practice mindful meditation, you do not need fancy clothes or candles, all you need is a few minutes and a place to be, without any distraction. The types are:

1. Four-four-eight breathing practices

This practice is a breathing technique. It is comparatively easy to practice even in the workplace and it can be done in just a few minutes.

How to practice?

- **Sit down:** And put yourself in a relaxed position. You can lay down on the floor or sit down on a chair by keeping your feet on the ground. It will only be helpful if you're completely at ease and comfortable.
- **Close your eyes:** Gradually and place your hands on your heart. Do not let yourself get distracted by the voices around. Rather go with them.
- **Breathe:** Start by breathing in through your nose for four counts of time. Fill your lungs with the fresh air to the point where you feel your body has expanded. And keep the count going.
- **Hold your breath:** In for four counts again. And note from where the air is passing. Whether it is going through the rib cage or stomach. In these counts, try to focus on your body and feel which parts of the body are tense and are in discomfort.

- **Breathe out:** Through your mouth for eight counts by making your lips pursed and creating a sound of whoosh. Without breaking the momentum, do it again for a count of four and repeat this technique three times in a row before feeling completely relaxed and mindful. The longer exhale keeps you calm in this technique. As you inhale, the blood pressure and heart rate increases, and your body parts get firm. Then, for every exhale the opposite happens. Breathing out for twice as long as breathing in, you're cutting off the wandering of the mind and bringing it back by focusing on your breath.

How is it helpful?

- This technique is very helpful in reducing stress levels and tension.
- It also helps to calm panic attacks and lowers heart rate.
- It also improves productivity working under pressure.
- It is also useful to avoid distractions.

2. Body scan mindful meditation

Our body goes through a lot. Sometimes alone by getting injured or sometimes it has to suffer because of mental distress. Most of the time we are aware of stiffness and pain in our body. But there are also some points when we cannot understand where the discomfort is. Body Scan Mindful Meditations allow us to feel our body deeply and helps us to trace all the pain we are carrying with ourselves. During the practice, we feel all the sensations and parts of our body thoroughly that often get neglected.

How to practice?

The body scan meditation can be done in both ways, while lying down, or sitting up. But mostly it is practiced by lying down on the floor.

These are the steps as follows:

- **Find a relaxed position:** The body scan begins with lying down on the back, while the palms are facing up and the feet are in a relaxed position and are apart from each other. You have to come out and lay on the floor for this.

- **Take a few deep breaths:** While lying still on the floor, without changing your position, breathe the air in through your nose and try to breathe from the belly rather than from the chest. As you breathe in and out, your abdomen will also expand and contract. Notice the air motion, Notice its rhythm, basically the process of breathing in and out. Keep your attention to the breath.

- **Feel your body:** Keep your focus on your body, how it is feeling, how the clothes are touching your body, try to feel the floor beneath you. Feel the warmth of your body. Feel the air around you. In this step, you have to be fully awake in the present to feel everything around you.

- **Scan your body:** Now, bring your attention to each of your body parts. Observe how each area feels. Start from your feet and toes, and then systematically move upward till you reach the top of your head. Observe the sensations moving upward. Try to note any pain and tension in those areas. Give attention to those parts where you do not feel any sensation or pain and gently try to breathe into them and feel them.

  If you feel tension and stiffness in any of the other parts, think of taking the pain from the part through your breath and leaving it in the air as you exhale. The body scan is to be fully aware of your bodily sensation in a mindful way. Doing this, your mind will get distracted by the other thoughts. What you have to do is to bring your attention back to your body. Be kind to yourself.

How is it helpful?

- Body scan mindful meditation helps in the reduction of inflammation and fatigue.

- It also controls hypertension (high blood pressure).
- It improves sleep intensity.
- Also, release the pain and distress.

3. Mindful walking

The core of mindful meditation is to observe our thoughts without trying to solve or hide them. Awareness comes after meditation helps accept the thoughts without reacting to them and makes us more mindful of the present.

This type of mindful meditation involves walking a few feet to lessen your stress level and soothe your nerves to perform well after coming back.

How to practice?

- **Come out for a walk for a few feet:** Come out and find a place where you can walk alone, it could be any street or just a less crowded area. No matter the form of Ambulation you use to go around is already making you more mindful, and it is an excellent technique for attention. Unless you keep yourself aware of the bodily sensations and keep your mind open to the voices around, you have done half of the work to become conscious of the present.

- **The pace of walking:** Keep your pace close to how you walk in everyday life. Do not try to rush and run to complete this 10-minute walking meditation. Keep your speed low.

  Just walk as you have been walking in your lobby in the afternoon.

- **See and hear:** Keep your eyes and ears open to see and hear all that is happening. Observe the streetlights and the pathway. Do not get drawn by the thoughts coming to your mind. But if you have, gently come back to the present and start noticing again. Your focus has to be on one thing; to calm and quieten your mind.

- **Feel your feet and ground:** Give time to your mind to be in the present time and it could be done by feeling your bodily sensation and its movement. Feel how your feet are touching the ground. First the heel, then your toe. How do your feet feel? What does the ground feel like? Is it soft or hard? Is it a tartan track or just a normal pathway or street? Starting from feet, move upwards gradually. Notice your leg movement, observe How your body shifts its balance as you put one foot in front of the other. Walk slowly and mindfully.

- **Breathe in the fresh air:** Noticing Breathing is also a great means of not getting lost in your thoughts. Breathe as you normally do but with consciousness. Now, bring your attention from body to breathing and see how the body expands as you breathe while walking. Breathe in slowly and now hold your breath for a few seconds and then release the air slowly again. Do it repeatedly and keep walking.

How is it helpful?

- Mindful walking is significant to the use of mini-break while working.
- It helps to strengthen your attention.
- It is also helpful in controlling your physical and emotional tension.
- Mindful walking is useful in managing stress and controlling negative energy.
- It also brings a feeling of wellbeing and improves physical health by controlling blood pressure and heart rate.

4. Loving-kindness meditation

Loving and having kindness for ourselves when we judge ourselves all the time is difficult. We get exhausted by constantly doubting ourselves, thinking about the past, and worrying about the future, basically not living in the time.

Loving-kindness is a self-care meditation that can help in improving our capability of self-acceptance and make us more compassionate towards others. Loving-kindness meditation is not a practice of achieving something rather it is just a practice to experience and attain utter happiness and good mental health. As we become more aware of meditation, we also learn how to be kind to ourselves.

What you need for this technique is a few minutes anywhere. This technique is very simple and effective to practice.

How to practice?

- **Relax:** Take a few minutes off from your busy life and set yourself in a comfortable place and just slow down your activity like you're about to do some sacred activity. Close your eyes, and relax your tensed parts of the body like shoulders, back, and head. Start by taking a few deep, long breaths. Try to create rhythm in your timing of breathing in and out and try to enjoy the delay in the process as you're holding the breath in for some time.
- **Feel yourself:** Bring your mind towards yourself. Imagine that you're breathing in inner peace and breathing out the tension and worry. Thank yourself for everything you do. Just try to be kind with your body and imagine it as

perfectly fine. Invite feeling of compassion to your body by reciting few phrases silently like;

May I be healthy,

May I be successful,

May I be safe,

May I be strong,

Keep your focus on one phrase at a time. Doing this, if your attention floats, be kind to your mind, and without criticizing yourself come back to repeating these phrases. Repeat three to four times these reassuring and positive phrases to yourself.

- **Imagine your loved ones:** Now move progressively from loving yourself to go giving compassion to others. So, to do that, imagine the people you love and who are very precious to you. They can be deceased ones. Imagine yourself as they are in front of you and you're giving them love and kindness. And saying these phrases to them individually.

May the person live long

May this person always be happy

May this person never go through distress

You can also send love to those with whom you are having any kind of problem. Extend your feelings of kindness and love for the people around the globe and imagine a connection between you two.

And finally, you can direct the feelings of love and compassion to the plants, animals, and universe itself.

How is it helpful?

- It helps boost self-love.
- It also helps in reducing stress.
- It also brings in a sense of positivity and reduces negative energy.

5. Mindful seeing and listening

The last technique of mindful meditation is mindful seeing and listening. These two mindful practices help in offering a break from giving full attention to self. Rather bring our notice to the surroundings.

This technique brings inner peace and breaks the preoccupation and judgment chain.

To practice mindful seeing exercise, you have to do nothing hard but to follow

How to practice? (Mindful seeing)

- **Go out and start looking around keenly:** There are many sights to observe and look at profoundly.
- **Find colors and shapes:** Notice everything that is present there but does not rush to name or count them. Rather go deep and focus on colors, patterns, shapes, and textures of those objects and over all things in the environment. Try to guess of their temperature, weight, and mass of the things too.

Be an observer. Think of yourself as a camera with a microscopic eye. Look at the sky, the clouds, the leaves, and how they are moving with air as you have to describe to a blind guy. Be an observer, not a scientist.

Drifting off. While observing, you will get distracted, and your mind will go wandering. But it is okay to happen. Softly pull your mind from those thoughts and continue focusing on the grass and any other thing in front of you.

How to practice? (Mindful listening)

- **Take a mini-break and sit comfortably:** Close your eyes calmly and start taking longer and deeper breaths to release all the stress and tension out.

- **Listen to the sounds:** Start by listening to the sounds of your breath as you are taking in the air. And keep listening to the voices around without reacting to them. The sounds can be of people around you, or the humming sounds of birds, or just dragging of chairs. You just have to listen to them as you completely cannot shut them off.

- **Notice:** You have to be present to listen keenly. Keeping your eyes close, try to make a guess of the sounds coming to your ears. If the sound is of a bird make a guess, whether it is of a sparrow or hummingbird.

Declutter: Practicing mindfulness, you have to declutter your head so you can fully focus on the moment.

You will get distracted and it will be hard to give full attention to the coming sounds. You will be taken away by the thoughts but whenever it happens with you, clear your head and bring your attention back to the listening.

How is it helpful?

- It improves attention span.
- It boosts positivity.
- It enhances productivity.
- It increases concentration level.

Chapter 2 - How to Calm Your Body and Mind

If we have to summarize the whole idea of meditation in a single phrase, we can say that meditation is a practice that quickly relaxes the body and calms the mind. An organism is made of both: body and mind. If the body is in a restless state, the mind will also not work properly. The same is the other way around. Both of them are connected as A healthy body has a sound mind.

So, to calm our body, we go for a warm bath, massages, and yoga. But how to calm our mind? Meditation calms the mind and which consequently relaxes the body too.

By being caught up in your busy mind, your body gets tired of it.

 So, when you feel drained out. Your mind feels tired after cluttering with hundreds of thoughts and it needs to be relaxed. The calmness can be brought back by doing this 5-minute sit-down meditation.

1. Find a comfortable place and position:

The first step is to set yourself in a place where you will be comfortable. You can be in your room, or a place outside. Where you will be less distracted. You can do this sitting up or lying down. And definitely, you don't need to be sitting by crossed legs.

2. Just Breathe:

Once you have found a good place and position. Now, Start breathing as this is the only job you're doing now. You don't have to make any efforts to control your breaths. You have to let them go in a general way, effortlessly.

3. Close your eyes and feel your body:

After doing this, what you have to do next is to just close your eyes and gradually start taking big, deep breaths, breathing in through the nose and out through the mouth. Just observe when inhaling that how your lungs fill the air, how your shoulders get tense, and how your body expands. Try to hold your breath for the count of three to five. And while exhaling, feel how lungs exhale the air through the stomach and mouth and how the body gets softened.

4. Accept what is happening around you:

Take a moment to just notice your surroundings without opening your eyes, feel the voices around and use this chance to get comfortable with all and just accept all the thoughts and voices.

5. Mind's wandering and controlling:

Very often, the mind wanders off and goes behind chasing a few thoughts, but when you realize, bring it back to feel the breath again.

6. Count to ten:

And as you bring your attention to the body, just start to become more aware of the movement of the breath, the rising and falling of the sensation. Try to examine your body parts. Feel where the stiffness and discomfort are. scan the complete body from head to toe. Do this thing thrice. Doing this, you might start thinking about other things, so just to make it easier to focus on breath, start counting the breath as they pass. Count one, as you feel the air filling your lungs, and count two, three, and four while holding your breath in. count five, as air goes out of the mouth, and so on. You can raise the count as you get comfortable with time. Repeat it a few more times.

7. Wrap it with gentleness:

And if you feel like opening your eyes, gently open them. In the meantime, before moving, just feel your mind and body. You will feel a lightness in your body and you will realize how much it was important to pause and take some time out.

A few minutes of activity is just a gateway to have better and positive behavior and relationships with yourself and others.

In this practice, feel how your feet and toes are touching the floor. At the end of the breathwork, just sit for 30 seconds and try to feel the surrounding serenity, the sounds, touch, and then slowly open your eyes.

Do this for five minutes and surely, this practice will fill the mind with freshness, and the body will also be at ease. Simply focus on your breath, feel the sensations in your body. If the mind wanders off, bring it back and again focus on the present moment. After doing this, you will feel your body calmer and mind relaxed.

Chapter 3 - Guided Meditation for Overcoming Anxiety, Stress, and Insomnia

Anxiety is a word we use to identify the fear that mostly has to do with the thought of a threat or something which will go wrong in the future, rather than in the present. Meditation is not the cure for these feelings. But a few pieces of research claim that when we create a little space between ourselves and what we are feeling or experiencing, our anxiety can calm and soften. If we react to things with a little amount of anxiety and stress, with time we will make a habit of it and it is very detrimental to our health. As a result, whenever we have to react, we will react in distress and with anxiety. This is why it is very essential to notice the difference between giving a reaction in the same manner to stress and anxiety and responding after learning how to react with mindfulness.

Guided Meditation to Overcome Anxiety

A guided meditation for anxiety is very helpful for both mild and severe anxiety.

How to practice?

- **Sitting comfortably:** Make sure you're sitting comfortably on the floor, having your legs crossed and back straight and tall. You are in a position where you are not only comfortable but also fully aware of your body. Where you can feel its sensation effectively. You are in a state Where neither you will get tired nor fall asleep. Resting your hands gently on your legs or whatever in position is most comfortable for you.

- **Closing your eyes:** If you like, allow your eyes to gently close or focus them on any object which is in front of you. It can be anything, a window or just a wall. Make sure you do not get drawn by it. You are just looking at it. Let yourself become as comfortable and relaxed as possible.

- **Breathing:** As you begin to settle in in this meditation, focus your attention on your breath. Feel the air moving through your nostrils as you simply let your breath continue to flow in and out ever so naturally and deliberately. You are not trying to change your breathing. You may want to just notice its pattern. And as you breathe, you are giving your attention to the air in your lungs as you slowly push your abdomen in and out along with your breath. Just gently focus on the natural rhythm of breathing and allow it to go deeper and let it bring relaxation for you. Your mind is probably getting distracted and wandering. Bring it back to the anchor of breathing.

- **Body scan:** Start to notice your body parts and feel if there is any tension. Notice your jaw, and if you feel any tension there, don't try to change it. Just simply breathe into the jaw and as you release the air, allow the tension to release a little too. Notice other parts of the body and feel the sensation in those parts. And if any muscle is tensed, try to release the tension with the exhale. You have to release any tension and tightness in your body as you exhale the air.

- **Speak the phrases to yourself:** Now as you are in relaxed mode, feeling pleasant and comfortable. Begin to speak some simple phrases to calm your anxiety or sense of panic.

When you begin, you may feel uncomfortable, perhaps a tightness in your chest or a rise in your heartbeat. And you want to quit it. But still, you have started. And as you continue doing it, you will feel your heartbeat getting settled and a great sense of inner calm and peace will softly come over you. and you are slowly detaching yourself from the ruminations and thoughts.

Start repeating the phrases to yourself. One after the other. It's your choice to speak them out loud like a lullaby or silently in your mind.

Give one complete breath pattern to each of these phrases and feel the immense energy of each of the words as you repeat them.

Continue to feel the air of your breath softly move in and out as you begin.

Now either out aloud or silently repeat the phrases.

As I am breathing in and out,

I am aware of my breath.

I am aware of my increased heartbeat.

I am fully aware of my body lying on the floor.

As I am breathing in and out,

I am aware of the anxiety within me.

I am aware that I am having sensations of panic.

I am aware of the chest tightness.

As I am breathing in and out,

I am aware of the negative thoughts within me.

But now I let go of all the negative thoughts.

Now I release them.

As I am breathing in and out

I calm my anxiety.

I calm my body.

I release the tightness in my chest.

I relax my mind.

I relax my body.

I slow down my thoughts.

As I am breathing in and out

I become free of my anxiety

And I find peace

And I find calm

As I am breathing in and out.

I am thankful to myself

I will be kind to myself

I will love myself

As I am breathing in and out

I let go of all.

I release everything.

I free myself from all.

- **Gently open your eyes and feel:** Now all the things have disappeared and dissolved. All the distress looks so meaningless. All the questions and worries that were giving you anxiety have become secondary and you have found what you are striving for.

- **Presence:** Being in the present, leaving the past behind, and Now you should feel a great sense of calm in your mind and body. You are now free, clear, present, and liberated.

  If you like to do this again, you can repeat these steps. To revise these phrases and reinforce them within you. But for now, take a few more moments to breathe in and out and relax in the moment of peace and stillness.

  Being fully aware, outer events have stopped affecting you and giving you anxiety and stress.

How is it helpful?

- It is helpful to decrease distress and control anxiety in critical situations.
- It helps to have a positive perspective on life.
- It also enhances self-awareness.

As human beings, stress and anxiety are natural parts of our lives. These feelings are not necessarily bad rather the problem is when we experience them so frequently, to the extent that they start to feel overwhelming. Firstly, we need to understand what stress is. Stress inherently is our thought about critical situations that confront us. There are two other major factors as well: first is what type of event happens to us, for example, an injury, a job loss, or overwork, and second is our response to the situation. But primarily it is our thought regarding our input in the critical situation. It is our mind which decides whether a situation is stressful or not. In a situation that outweighs our abilities, we think of it as stressful and if we think our skills are better than what the situation demands, we don't see the situation as stressful. We tend to run away from these thoughts and feelings because we tend to think that they will cause us harm and pain and that will only intensify the feelings of hopelessness. Our assessment and response to the situation are often influenced by our past experiences especially our traumatic and stressful experiences. Stress can activate from any kind of situation. Our thoughts make us feel anxious, fearful, angry, and frustrated most of the time. Two people will never respond in the same way to given situations and it depends on the individual's skills, perception, and past experience not on the situation.

When things do not work out the way we want them to be, we become frustrated and anxious. A feeling of ill will comes to our mind and we start having resentment for the things. But if we accept and realize the situation, changing how we look at the situation can be very helpful.

As it is said, most of our stress comes from our thinking. Very often, stress lies inside. It is part of normal life. Stress is good in a small proportion. It motivates us. It also helps us to be more productive and useful. But stress is harmful if we strongly show a response to it. It is the way that we approach life. It is the way we teach our minds. It is the outlet of all the frustration of not getting what we think was necessary. If we learn about ourselves and our reaction to stressful situations, we can also learn to handle the repercussions of stress more effectively. This is what stress management is. It is not about avoiding stress rather it is about how calmly we respond to a stressful situation. Furthermore, if we begin to work differently with our mind and if we can change our perspective to the negative or stressful thoughts that arise in our mind. If we learn to see things differently when such feelings arise, this could change not only how we feel internally but the way we meet others as well. With meditation, it is possible to do so.

Studies have shown that meditation is really helpful in increasing our ability to deal with stress.

To reduce the stress, a meditation technique called "Noting" is introduced here. It is primarily helpful when we are constantly getting drawn by and distracted by the thoughts of stress and anxiety. While meditating, sometimes our mind wanders off and we do not know how to react to the situation. Here noting technique helps by giving us a very clear direction and a sense of clarity and confidence. In the moment of noting, we pause and try to identify the kind of distraction. We note either we were distracted by the thoughts or feelings. Noting the nature of distraction is almost like dealing with the distraction and it is quite helpful in letting go of any distraction and gently come back to the object of focus. The mind will get distracted again and what will we do? We will simply practice the same approach. We will note the kind of distraction and it will become quite easy to deal with the distraction. With gentle acknowledgment, we only need to note the distraction when we come to realize that we were swept away with the thoughts. After the acknowledgment, we effortlessly return to the object of focus.

How to practice?

The technique aims is to make more space in the mind, to make it less judgmental and less reactive. A mind that allows you to be more "a present being" and less stressed.

- **Find a conducive environment:** Find a comfortable seated position. Cross your legs or kneel just make sure that you are sitting comfortably. Now gently close your eyes or if you don't want to do that for now, you can maintain a slight, soft and relaxed focus. You have to just sit in a position where you will not get physically distracted during the meditation.
- **Shift attention inward:** Start taking longer and deeper breaths, in and out through the nose.
  Allow the weight of breath to bring you into the present. Rest your attention on the anchor of the breath and start to notice, as you breathe in, how your lungs fill with air. Give attention to the texture and quality of the breath. As you breathe out each time, notice how your muscles get softened in your body. As you are breathing in and out, slightly start closing your eyes and stop for a moment and enjoy that feeling of stillness and being stopped. Take a couple of more deep breaths and let everything outside of the breath disappear, to go out of focus, like a little retreat. Feel how your body feels while breathing: is there a

sense of heaviness or lightness? Is there a sense of tension or stillness? You are just noticing, not trying to solve or hide it. You are getting more aware of your space each time you breathe in and out.

- **Focus:** With all the thoughts in your mind, you do not have any object of focus rather you are aware of everything around you. There must be sounds. You do not have to show any resistance to them. Just allow them to come and go. Thoughts are also coming and going and you just have to let them without any resistance.

- **The mind will get distracted:** In this practice, your mind will get distracted and attention will be drawn away. Your Mind will drift away from the path of breathing. But in this practice, it will be helpful. Be gentle and kindly note what the thought is. If the mind is worried about to-do lists, you just have to gently repeat the word "planning" in your mind and return your attention to the anchor of breath.

You may notice, during meditation, the mind will revert back to what happened in past days. You could put those thoughts in the category of "past".

- **Note all the thoughts and emotions that are coming to distract you:** You may notice, during meditation, the mind will be worried about the presumptions. You could simply put the label of "future" on those thoughts as you notice them. And the mind gets distracted by the things you don't know how to categorize, just simply put the label of "don't know". Mind is not only keep thinking about thoughts, rather there is emotional equality. Sometimes we think about a conversation and find it joyous. Sometimes we get angry or frustrated over the words of others. While in meditation, our mind gets caught up in those emotions. When you note that the mind is distracted by those conversations, try to identify the emotion and bring the attention back to the breath. The drifting of mind has no limit. You could spend the whole meditation chasing after the mind by noting its distractions. So, it is okay if the mind cannot stop distractions, you just have to keep doing the practice to cultivate your mindful and de-stressed vision. When you realize you have been distracted, but now you have come back and you are not involved in those thoughts anymore where there was lots of criticism and judgment. You can note bodily sensations and feel how your body is pressed against the seat or floor. Your breathing is an alternative object of focus. Then note the coming sounds of the surroundings without showing any subjectivity or resistance. Now allow your mind to be completely free.

After a few more breaths, gently open your eyes and appreciate the feeling of having stopped being completely still. This is the center of meditation. So, you gently acknowledge it and bring your attention back to the breathing again. With this belief that the peace of mind that you are looking for is already here.

So, the takeaway here is rather than fighting to clear out the stressed and unpleasant feelings, acknowledging and accepting them during the ongoing stressful situation is really crucial.

It is not a practice to learn to be more present rather it is about changing our perspective to the experiences, changing how we relate to them. Being less judgmental and less critical of not only ourselves but also of those who are around us. When we bring these points into use, we become less stressed.

How is it helpful?

- During a stressful situation, the practice of noting technique helps in reducing the stress response.
- It helps reduce stress hormone levels.
- It is also helpful in reducing blood pressure.

Stress and anxiety not only affect our mental health but our physical health also suffers in these situations. Due to stress and anxiety, the tension in our muscles increases. This can lead to the stiffness of the body or even pain in the spine or neck. Progressive muscle relaxation helps us to become more aware of the tension so we can better identify and address it. PMR involves the repeated tightening and relaxing of different muscle groups. This technique holds the theory that when we are physically relaxed, we cannot be anxious or stressed. Deep relaxation has proved to be quite effective during critical situations including anxiety, stress, insomnia, and high blood pressure. PMR has successfully participated in the treatment of health problems, including anxiety, and stress. PMR is not only effective for releasing the tension from the muscles of the body rather it has a strong impact on the mind as well.

How to practice?

The thought behind this technique is to intentionally tense one group of muscles and then to release the tension. So, before you begin, there are four basic steps that you need to keep in mind while practicing this technique. The first is to create tension, the second is to relax the tensed muscle, the third is to give rest to the relaxed muscle, and the fourth is to start again with a different group of muscles.

- **Find a quiet place:** Find a quiet and free from distractions place for the next fifteen to twenty minutes. Lie down on the floor or recline in a chair. Get rid of any physical distractions. Sit comfortably in a cross-legged position and erect your back by leaning back the shoulders. Place your hands on your lap. If you're sitting on a chair, just upright your back and place your hands on the arms of the chair.

- **Take a few slow even breaths:** Now, after being comfortable start taking deeper and longer breaths. Breathe in through your nose and breathe out through your mouth. Take a breath from your abdomen as you count to three. As you breathe in, feel the rise of your stomach. After a short pause, exhale calmly by counting to three again. Feel the fall of your stomach as you breathe out. Continue this practice for three to five minutes until you feel relaxed.

- **Contract one muscle group:** As you breathe in, contract the muscle group in your toes by waving them into your feet. Tense the muscles hard but not to the point of pain and hold the tension for three to ten seconds. Feel the tension in your toes and try to tense only one muscle group at one time. After holding, release the tension slowly from your toes and let them relax. Give yourself ten to twenty seconds to relax, before moving to the next muscle group. Notice how the muscles feel when they are tense and how they feel when they are relaxed.

- **Move upward:** Now, move to the next muscle group which is the legs. Slowly increase the tension in your calves and quadriceps. Then try to tense the muscles as hard as possible without causing any discomfort or pain and do this for a good thirty seconds. After doing it, notice the tension is melting away as you slowly relax them. During the practice, keep breathing slowly and deeply.

- Now come to the next muscle group: buttocks. Press your buttocks together tightly and hold the tension for over fifteen seconds. Then while you exhale, fully relax your muscles and focus on changing sensations.

- Now squeeze your stomach. Take a deep breath and hold it for ten to fifteen seconds and suck into a tight knot too. Then slowly release the tension from your mouth. Take ten to twenty seconds to relax your tensed muscles.

- Moving gradually upwards, arch your back up and take it away from the chair's support or the floor. As you breathe in, gently create tension in that particular muscle group and hold it for ten seconds. With the exhale, fully relax your tensed muscles. Notice the feelings before and after the relaxation. You will feel that muscles will become softer and lighter. Then take a break for ten seconds to relax the muscle.

- After that comes the muscles of the chest. After breathing, you have to hold the breath for ten to fifteen seconds in that muscle area and slowly release the breath from your mouth. Take a good ten to fifteen minutes to relax after the release of the breath and notice the change after tensing your muscle.

- The next muscle for tension is the muscles of the neck. First, with breathing in, create tension in the front of the neck by touching your chest with your chin for five to ten seconds. Keep one thing in mind, leave the muscle when you start feeling the pain. Now slowly release the tension as you exhale. Rest for ten seconds before creating tension in the back of the neck. And for this, you need to press the back of your head against your support. It can be a floor or a chair headrest. Do it for ten minutes and as you breathe out, slowly release your neck from the tension and bring it back to the prior position. Give your muscles a rest for the next ten seconds and try to feel the relaxation after the tension there.

- Now tense your lips. After giving rest to your neck, breathe the air in through your nose and tightly press your lips together as you hold the air in your lungs. Slowly release the tension from your lips as you breathe the air out from your mouth at the same time. Give the muscles rest for a good five minutes and move to the next muscle group.

- After lips, tense your cheeks and jaws. Tense the muscles in your cheeks and jaws and smile as widely as possible for you. Do it for ten seconds. Then slowly release the tension with the breath and after that, put your cheeks and jaw for relaxation.

- Now, tense your eyes by closing them as tightly as it is possible. If you are wearing contact lenses, remove them before tensing your eyes to avoid any harmful conditions. Close the eyes for fifteen seconds and slowly open them with the exhalation. Now give them a rest for a few seconds more.

- And move to the forehead. Squeeze the muscles in your forehead and wrinkle them into a tense frown. Hold it for fifteen seconds and feel the muscles as they become tighter and tenser. Then, slowly release the tightness in your forehead as slowly as you can. Try to notice the difference before and after the tightness of the muscles. With this, Keep breathing in a slow and ever manner.

- After the basic muscle contraction, now its shoulders turn. What you have to do to increase tension in your shoulders is simply raise your shoulders up towards the ears and shrug them. Hold the tension for fifteen seconds. With the exhale, release the tension from your shoulders and let them relax for the next few seconds.

- Come to the arms. First, you need to make a fist of your hands and bend both of your arms at the elbow as you are flexing your biceps and triceps. Do it for ten to fifteen seconds and create as much tension there as it is possible to create without any discomfort. After holding, release the tension slowly and calmly by breathing evenly along.

- Here comes the turn of wrists. As you breathe in, stretch your hands and bend them back at the wrist. Hold this tensed position for ten seconds and as you breathe out, release the tension with the air. Give your arms and hands a quiet rest of ten seconds.

- At last, the hands. Clench your hands and make a fist. After creating the tension, keep it for fifteen seconds and then slowly release as you release the air out from your mouth.

How is it helpful?

- The progressive muscle relaxation technique helps to lessen stress.
- PMR helps to relieve anxiety.

- Along with that, PMR helps to reduce blood pressure among people with heart disease.
- People who are dealing with insomnia argue that practicing PMR at night helps them to fall asleep and this technique also improves their quality of sleep.

PMR is an excellent technique to learn about the body and how it is reacting to certain situations. With practice and time, you can correctly identify the signs of stress and tension in your body and you can deal with it more mindfully.

Insomnia is a prevalent sleep disorder. As sleep is a very necessary factor of our overall health and well-being. Due to insomnia, we have difficulty with sleep. It becomes hard for us to have an adequate amount of quality sleep. Lack of sleep adversely impacts our physiological health and daily productivity. Hyperarousal is another very potent factor of insomnia and it is caused by stress. It badly affects the harmony between sleep and wakefulness.

Research suggests that Meditation helps to improve insomnia. Meditation forms a relaxed state of mind which is conducive to make you fall asleep. When we are stressed or anxious, our mind stays hyperactive and we find difficulty with having sleep. Meditation teaches us to relax and be more aware of the present.

How to practice?

- **Find a quiet place:** When meditating before bedtime and in your room, remove all the distractions. Switch your phone off. Turn the light off. Lie down in a comfortable position. Be in a position where you won't be physically distracted for the next few minutes. Close your eyes.

- **Take big, deep breaths:** As you are in a comfortable position, now start taking longer, deeper breaths. Breathe in through your nose and breathe out through your mouth. Inhale for 10 counts from your nose slowly. Then hold your breath for 10 counts. After holding the breath, exhale for 10 counts. You need to repeat this breathing exercise five to ten times. Notice how your lungs fill with air and your body expands, as you breathe in. Notice how your stomach and chest rise as you hold the breath inside. Notice how your body softens as you breathe out through your mouth. Hold your focus on your breathing throughout the session of meditation.

- **Close your eyes:** While keeping your focus on the breath, gently close your eyes and pay attention to your surroundings. Notice the sounds of silence around you. Shift your focus on the awareness of the surroundings. You do not have to actually identify the sounds coming to your ears, you just have to let them come and go. Your only aim of this meditation is to be present and acknowledge whatever is happening around you. You have to be aware and present.

- **Be focused:** While meditating, there is the highest possibility of mind wandering at night time. The mind wanders at night the most because you are not involved in any physical activity and your body is still and at rest. When you realize, your mind has drifted away, just gently bring it back to focus on your breath.

- **Feel your body:** Now, shift your focus from your surroundings to your body now. Try to feel all the bodily sensations and movements. Try to find the feelings of heaviness or lightness in the body. Try to find the feelings of restlessness or stillness in your body. Try to sense how the body feels. With that, notice where in the body you feel the movement, the rising and falling sensations of the breath. Keep all of your focus on the awareness of your breath and on your bodily movements on inhaling, holding, and exhaling the air.

- **Be calm:** Keep breathing in big deep breaths and just let all the thoughts go away for a couple of more minutes. Try to let all the tensions and worries fade away as you are not trying to hold them at all. Try to calm your tense and anxious nerves and gently remind them that you are bigger than your problems. Remind yourself that now, in this time, nothing matters. You are free and relaxed. You are not bound to any thought. Take a few more breaths and gently open your eyes. Before getting up, just sit for a few more minutes and appreciate the calmness and relaxation in your body. Appreciate your free mind. Appreciate your breath which helped you calm your body and mind. Appreciate the awareness you are having now. Appreciate the lightness. And after doing this, if you want to go to bed you can. Just try to be in an aware mood till you fall asleep.

How is it helpful?

- Meditation helps to improve the efficiency and quality of sleep.
- It helps to calm your body and prepare your mind to sleep.
- It improves your coping mechanism during stressful situations as your mind has rested as you were asleep.

Chapter 4 - Affirmations to Overcome Anxiety, Stress and for Deep Sleep

Affirmations are simple statements. It is a small set of positive words that are usually direct to ourselves to promote self-love and care and eliminate worry and anxiety. Positive affirmations produce the feel-good hormones in our brain, as we recite them to ourselves. The more we repeat them, it is more likely to believe that the hormones will start changing our thought pattern and our mind will accept them as facts with time. It has been proved that the daily use of affirmation has been an ally in making our minds work more positively.

Positive affirmations to overcome anxiety

- Start from shorter statements, you can create your own personally meaningful statements too.
- I breathe in peace and I breathe out tension.
- I am safe at this moment.
- I am in control.
- I am calm and relaxed.
- I am full of loving and positive energy.
- I am strong and well-aware.
- I am thankful for the blessings.

- I am opening up to feel inner peace.
- I am learning to overcome my fears and anxiety.
- I am able to eliminate negativity from my mind.
- I am able to fill my mind with positive energy.
- I am able to control my mind and body.
- I am completely fine right now.
- I am freeing myself from stress and anxiety.
- I have the ability to overcome my anxiety.
- I have everything to have a happy life.
- All is well in my small world.

Positive Affirmations to have a peaceful sleep

You get anxious and stressed during your daily routine and it hurts your night sleep as well. Using positive affirmations can change your mindset and can also solve the problem of sleepless nights. There is nothing more refreshing than waking up in the morning after having a good sleep.

So, to get that sleep, giving 5 to 10 minutes to this activity you need to repeat a few affirmations to yourself. You can also put your hand on your belly or heart as a self-comforting mechanism. These affirmations have to sound true to you and you can coax yourself into a restful sleep. You can change them anytime.

- As I breathe in and out
- I let go of all of my worries and tension

- I let go of all of my stress.
- I let go of all the negative energy and I invite positive energy.
- I am calm and relaxed
- I am at peace and everything is fine.
- I am grateful for the blessing and challenges in my life.
- I am having a mindful day.
- I am learning to be mindful.
- I forgive all, and I have no regrets and grudges.
- I am happy to sleep and will have a great day tomorrow.
- I am ready to face everything with positivity.
- I am going to make my coming life beautiful and will forget my past life.
- I am healing through sleep.
- I am ready to fall asleep now.

You can repeat these phrases to yourself whenever you need the confirmation and love to go through the day and have peaceful sleep at night. You have to stand true to yourself while saying these affirmations to yourself and you will see the big changes by small words.

Chapter 5 - Guided Meditation for Sweet Relaxation for Deep Sleep

Nearly one in five people sometimes have trouble with sleeping. There are multiple reasons. Stress and anxiety are potent factors behind having sleeping difficulty. These feelings do not allow our body and mind to wind up and fall asleep. Our body reacts actively to stressful conditions. Our muscles get tense and stiff and constant muscle tension can consequently affect our health badly including, headaches and heart problems. Our sleeping cycle gets affected and in return, it affects our hormone balance, our blood pressure, and overall physical health. It is not possible to sleep with a mind which is constantly chattering and a body that is tensed and disturbed.

So, relaxation techniques are genuine assistance in the management of stress. These techniques not only help in winding up the thoughts but also enhance our sleep quality. There are numerous relaxation meditations and they work differently for every person. Some relaxation techniques have already been discussed in this book.

- **Progressive muscle relaxation (PMR):** It is a technique in which we tense our body parts from head to toe. There is tension, hold, the release of tension, and relaxation of the muscle group. It is very helpful in relaxing the body.it is just a 10 to 15 minutes activity.

- **Full body scan:** This technique is a mindful exercise to identify any distress, or pain in the body. In this meditation, we thoroughly notice every part of the body. We try to feel every sensation and movement in the body. Even from breathing, we notice lungs. We notice how the chest rises and falls, as we breathe in and out.

- **Sight and sound meditation:** This technique is also very helpful to free your mind from the marathon of thoughts. These two sensory activities help to maintain focus on the present. We try to focus on what we are seeing in the present time and what we are hearing in the now.

- **Deep Breathing:** The breathing technique is almost used in every meditation. Breathing is a very potent element of every relaxation meditation. In deep breathing, we tend to take a breath in from our nose as long as possible. We have to hold the breath in our stomach for the longest time. Then, we exhale the breath from our mouth. This technique is helpful to release the tension from our bodies. It also works as an object of focus in many meditations to control the wandering of the mind.

The following techniques are very helpful for sweet relaxation for sleep.

1. Imagery Relaxation

Imagery relaxation or visualization is a form of meditation in which you use your imaginations to create a state in your mind that's pleasant, peaceful, and relaxing.

The use of imagination is an efficient way to stop the busy mind. So to overcome the feelings of unhappiness and stress, divert your mind to a positive and pleasant image. The practice asks you to create an image in your mind which you find peaceful and calm. The image can be from your past experiences or it can also be futuristic. It is helpful to prevent your mind from getting stuck in negative and worrisome thoughts.

How to practice?

- **Take deep breaths:** Before starting the meditation, it is important to be in a quiet place and lie down in a comfortable position for the next few minutes to not be get disturbed by any physical distraction. After doing this, close your eyes and start taking deep breaths. Breathe in from your nose. Hold the breath for a few seconds in your chest. Breathe out through your mouth. Keep doing this practice throughout this whole meditation.

- **Feel your body:** Quickly scan your body. Notice if there is any tension or stiffness in any muscle of the body and if it is there, try to relax it. Notice the sensations as you breathe in and out. Let your body get soft against the bed as you move further in this meditation.

- **Mind-wandering:** Your night is not used to being quiet. It is always chattering and cluttering. It is almost impossible to make it stop. So, during meditation too, your mind will go wandering and chasing thoughts. It is completely fine because you cannot stop it from happening. So, when you realize that your mind is occupied just simply bring it back into what you are doing.

- **Imagine:** As you have closed your eyes, now start imagining yourself in a peaceful place. Create a very vivid picture in your mind. Incorporate as many sensory details as possible. It is important to see the sight, hear the sounds, feel the touch and smell the scent. For instance, imagine yourself amidst a forest, with green tall trees around you, a clear blue sky, and dreamy clouds movement. You can hear the air whistles and birds' voices. You can feel the breeze on your face. You can feel the warmth of the sun as well. You can feel the hard muddy road. As you continue along the road, breathing in and out, you can clearly see the stream of clear and shiny water and the sound of water running is coming to your ears mildly. You can smell the pine trees and the scent of different wildflowers. You are walking calmly without any worry or tension. There is nothing holding you back. You are enjoying your time there in the forest as you always wanted to come here. You can keep imagining until sleep arrives.

- **Relax:** Enjoy the feelings of being free and lighted as you explore the pleasant place. When you feel ready, you can gently open your eyes and come to "the now" and the present. Take a moment before getting up, and feel your mind and body's calmness.

The more you will practice, the more you will be able to imagine better and for a longer time. Practice this imagery relaxation practice regularly for ten to fifteen minutes before going to bed.

How is it helpful?

- It helps in relaxing the body which lowers the blood pressure and balances the hormones.
- It enhances the quality of sleep, and with that, it also enhances the quality of life.

2. The Military Method

The popular military method would be very efficient to make you fall asleep within two minutes, regardless of how stressed you are. The military method was used by combat pilots to fall asleep quickly with all the distractions of gunfire behind them.

This practice usually takes just 120 seconds to complete. This practice is also helpful for those who have to sleep by sitting up. You will also find this practice helpful no matter how anxious and stressed you would be.

How to practice?

It is just a four-step method.

- **Be comfortable:** Bring yourself in the most relaxed and comfortable position. Lie down on your bed. It is better to lie on your back as it is helpful for the relaxation of the muscles. Turn the lights off and switch your phone off to avoid any physical distraction. Start breathing slowly and deeply.

- **Relax the face:** Relaxing your face is the main factor of this meditation. Relax your entire face, every muscle, including jaws, tongue, head, forehead, cheeks, and muscles around your eyes. Remove any kind of tension from your head and also from your facial muscles. While relaxing your muscles, gently close your eyes. Feel the muscles in your face getting relaxed and limp. When your face is relaxed and limp, a signal goes to your body informing it that all is set to sleep. Notice how your breath is getting slow and deep.

- **Release of the tension:** Now moving towards relaxing the body, drop your shoulders as low as possible as if they are falling toward your feet. Put your neck in a relaxed position. Breathe in from your nose and breathe out through your nose slowly and evenly.

  Now drop your arms. Start by loosening the upper arm, then the lower arm on one side. Then do the same to the other arm. Along with that, keep breathing in and breathing out slowly to relax your upper part of the body and especially your chest.

  Now remove any tension from your thighs, calves, and legs orderly.

- **Clear the mind:** Now your body is fully relaxed and limp, it is time to relax your mind for ten seconds to fall asleep. To relax the mind, imagine a serene scene as you are lying in the bottom of a canoe on a lake and a very clear blue sky is visible. Or imagine lying in a black hammock in a dark room. If these two sleep-producing fantasies don't work for you, try repeating the phrase "don't think", "don't think", "don't think" over and over again for ten seconds. And within ten seconds, you will fall asleep.

This technique was given in a book by Sharon Ackerman. The pilots practiced it for six weeks and it worked for them.

How is it helpful?

- This technique is an effective way of falling asleep within just two minutes.
- It improves our sleeping cycle and consequently our overall physical and mental health.

3. Autogenic Relaxation

The autogenic technique is a widely used relaxation technique. This technique uses the power of the mind to relax the body. It is quite similar to progressive muscle relaxation, but there is no need to contract any muscle. Instead, you influence and decrease muscle tension by repeating a few phrases consciously as you scan your whole body thoroughly.

This term means" coming from within". This skill focuses on the feelings of heaviness, breath, and the feelings of warmth in the body. The feelings of heaviness are a sign of your muscles' relaxation and warmth is a sign of blood flow. Both sensations are positive indicators of relaxation of the body.

How to practice?

- **Find a quiet place for twenty minutes:** After being in a quiet place, sit or lie down in a comfortable position to avoid any physical disturbance. Allow your body to relax and calm. Let the feelings of warmth and heaviness naturally rise from your body. Do not force it.

- **Breathe and relax your body:** Take a deep breath from your nose and hold it for two seconds and then breathe out. As you breathe out, let all the worries and tension leave your body. Keep breathing slowly and gently. Allow your body to relax as you breathe in and out. As you are breathing, allow your eyes to get close. Your breath is becoming smoother and slower. Now repeat these phrases to yourself,

  "My breath is slow. My breath is smooth"

  "My breath is slow. My breath is smooth"

  "My breath is slow. My breath is smooth"

  as you breathe, your body relaxes with you. Each breath is drawing out the tension from your body and leaving it soft and relaxed. Your body feels calm and relaxed.

- Now concentrate on your arms, first your right arm. Say these words to yourself three times. "My right arm is heavy. My left arm is warm." And feel the warmth and heaviness throughout your arms as you are lying relaxed on the grass and the sun is shining.

- Allow all of the tension to flow from right arm to left arm. Repeat these lines to yourself three times.

  > "My Left arm is heavy. My left arm is warm".

  > "My Left arm is heavy. My left arm is warm".

  > "My Left arm is heavy. My left arm is warm".

- Feel the heaviness in both of your arms. Repeat these phrases to both of your arms.

  > "My both arms are heavy. My both arms are warm"

  > "My both arms are heavy. My both arms are warm"

  > "My both arms are heavy. My both arms are warm"

  Now, they have released all of the holding tension and now they are fully relaxed and warm under the shiny sun.

- While your arms are relaxed, scan your body from head to toe and try to find if there is any tensed muscle. Make your shoulder relax, your jaws relax and your mind free.

- Now all the tension has been flown to the neck and back muscles. Feel the heaviness and warmth in your back and neck muscles and repeat these words.

> "My neck and back are heavy. My neck and back are warm".

> "My neck and back are heavy. My neck and back are warm".

> "My neck and back are heavy. My neck and back are warm".

As you repeat these words, you feel your back and neck are getting free from all the tension and stiffness. Contract your muscles of back and neck and after holding the contraction, release slowly. As with the warmth of the sun, your whole upper body, including your arms, shoulders, face, neck, and back is feeling warm and heavy. You are breathing deeply and smoothly. Your body is relaxed and calm. Your heart is beating evenly and calmly.

- Now, feel your right leg as it is tensed and repeat these words,

> "My right leg is heavy. My right leg is warm".

> "My right leg is heavy. My right leg is warm".

> "My right leg is heavy. My right leg is warm".

Feel as the tension from your right leg has disappeared and it is now fully relaxed and warm.

- Turn your attention to your left leg and notice if there is tension. After noticing, repeat the phrases in your mind. Repeat the phrases.

    "My left leg is heavy. My left leg is warm".

    "My left leg is heavy. My left leg is warm".

    "My left leg is heavy. My left leg is warm".

- Now feel both of your legs warm and heavy as all the tension has been released. Now say, "I am relaxed and comfortable.

    "My both legs are heavy. My both legs are warm".

    "My both legs are heavy. My both legs are warm".

    "My both legs are heavy. My both legs are warm".

Imagine yourself lying on the soft grass with fully heavy and warm legs.

- Now draw your attention toward both of your arms and both of your legs. And say the phrases.

    "My both arms and legs are heavy. My both arms and legs are warm"

    "My both arms and legs are heavy. My both arms and legs are warm"

"My both arms and legs are heavy. My both arms and legs are warm"

Continue to imagine yourself lying on the soft grass with fully warm arms and legs.

- Continue to breathe in and out slowly and smoothly. Now notice your forehead and try to free it from all the lingering thoughts. Try to cool and calm it down. Free yourself from your mind for a few moments. Repeat these words 3 times.

"I am relaxed and calm.

My arms are warm and heavy.

My legs are warm and heavy.

My arms and legs are warm and heavy.

My breathing is smooth.

My forehead is cool."

- Lastly, bring your attention to your heart, and release all the tension from it and make its blood flow calm and even. Repeat these phrases 3 times.

"I am relaxed and calm.

My arms are warm and heavy.

My legs are warm and heavy.

My arms and legs are warm and heavy.

My breathing is smooth.

My forehead is cool

My heartbeat is calm and even"

So, as you wind up the exercise, take deep breaths and if you feel any tension, release it and slowly open your eyes and feel the energy inside. Feel the alertness and awareness inside you. Feel relaxed and calm and try to be in this state for a few moments to experience it completely. And you will already feel yourself half asleep, as all of your muscles are resting.

How is it helpful?

- It helps in the cure of chronic migraines.
- It helps in the disease of blood vessels.
- It also helps to control blood pressure.

4. Self-Hypnosis

Hypnosis is a Greek word that means sleep. It is quite similar to sleep but in hypnosis, we do not completely lose our sense of awareness. We respond to things and senses. We have experienced hypnosis multiple times. Daydreaming, remembering a past event, or watching tv, all these are hypnotic states.

In this relaxation meditation, there will be positive thoughts and images to relax and destress ourselves. It is about experiencing our own thoughts. Self-hypnosis is quite similar to progressive muscle relaxation. Muscle relaxation puts our body in a hypnotic state. It means we are relaxed and open to any kind of suggestive conditions. As we are relaxing our tense and stressed body to fall asleep, it is important to use a keyword or a phrase that is opposite to our problem. It is the goal of hypnosis. For example, if our problem is anxiety, our keyword should be "calm and relaxed" or "now I am relaxed".

How to practice?

- **Find a comfortable place:** Find a quiet place where you won't get physically distracted for the next few minutes. Lie down in a comfortable position where your body can relax and limp.

- **Take deep breaths:** As you are lying in a comfortable position, start breathing deeply and slowly. Breathe in from your nose and as the air goes in, hold it in your abdomen and then exhale the air from your mouth. Taking breaths, close your eyes, and put your all attention into breathing. Breathe, and notice how your lungs fill the air and how stiff and tense your body is. As you exhale, notice how your body gets softened and muscles relax. Keep your focus on breathing in and breathing out. You are slowly moving towards the hypnotic state.

- **Relax your muscles:** Start relaxing your muscles one by one. Relax your body keeping the three points in your mind: contract the muscle, release the tension, relax the muscle. Start from the lower part of the body. As you are relaxing your muscle, repeat the phrases about the muscle you're relaxing.

At first, tense your feet and toes. Tense them for 3 seconds and repeat the phrases,

"heavier and warmer. Relaxed and calmed".

Now release the tension slowly and put the particular muscle for relaxing and keep breathing deeply.

After that, moving to legs muscles. Tense the muscles of the thighs, calves, and legs. Keep the tension for a few seconds and repeat the phrase "heavier and warmer", 3 times and relax it slowly with your breath. Saying the phrase "relaxed and calmed".

Now move towards your upper body, contract the muscles of the chest and stomach. Hold the tension and say the phrase, "heavier and heavier" and as you release the tension, repeat the phrase," relaxed and calmed".

Now create tension in your back and neck muscles. Create tension and after holding the tension, release it by saying, "relaxed and calmed", "loosen and calmed". Repeat them 3 to 4 times.

Tense the muscles of arms and shoulders, hold the tension as long as it is possible, and then release as you exhale the air with saying these phrases three times. "relaxed and drooping", "calmed and composed"

Bring the tension in your facial muscles, including your jaw, your eyes, your cheeks, and your tongue. And smile as widely as you can to create the tension. Then release the tension and repeat these phrases too.

"Smooth and relaxed", "loosen and calmed". Repeat these key phrases three times as you inhale and exhale.

Now lastly, bring tension in your forehead muscles and hold it. As you exhale the tension with the air, repeat the key phrase, "smooth and relaxed, calm and composed". Now your body is fully relaxed and prepared to be in a hypnotic state.

- **A place to imagine:** As you're breathing deeply and slowly. Your body is also relaxed and calm. There is no physical or mental distraction. Start to imagine your favorite place. Your favorite place can be any place, for instance, it can be a park behind your home or a mountain or a beach. Start by imagining your journey to your favorite place. Count your steps by counting numbers with that. As you take one step, count 1. As you take the next step you feel more relaxed and calmed. Each count is deepening the tranquility in you. You are counting and taking steps. Now from far, you can see your favorite place. As you are approaching your favorite place, you are feeling deeply relaxed. Now you have reached and you are standing at your favorite place. Look around and see the things. The colors. The shapes. The textures and the beauty. Listen to the sounds. Smell the scent. Taste the air. Feel the calmness. If your favorite place is the beach. Imagine as you can listen to the sounds of waves, the hiss of the foam. Imagine as you are seeing and hearing the seagulls. Imagine as the sun is so warm and shiny. There is direct light on you and it is making you feel warmer. There is water and sand under your feet. You can feel as the water goes through them. You can feel the wet sand. Involve and incorporate all of your senses: sounds, smell, touch, and taste. Imagine vividly and clearly.

- **Repeat these suggestions:** Now consciously repeat these suggestions until you feel completely calm. You can alter them as well and if you want to make personal suggestions, you can also do that.

I am drifting deeper and deeper

I am feeling peace and calmness

I am going down and down into total tranquility

I am drifting deep into complete calmness

I am hovering on the relaxation.

Coming out of the hypnotic state. When you feel you have spent enough time in your favorite place, and you want to come back. Don't leave the meditation in between. Rather coming out of the hypnotic state is equally important as coming into the hypnotic state. So, to start, start counting in backward order from 10 to 1, and in between the numbers, remind yourself that you are becoming more relaxed, more calmed, more alert, fresher, and more conscious. As you reach number 2, gently open your eyes. As you say number 1, finally recall the phrases of being fully awake and alert, being fully calm and relaxed. With the completion of the technique, your body was half asleep because muscles were fully relaxed. It is the most inducing state to fall asleep.

It is okay if you are not getting successful at creating an image or holding it for a longer time. Self-hypnosis will get better with practice. During this relaxation meditation, don't let your mind drift away. And keep its focus on your visit to your favorite.

How is it helpful?

- It has a positive impact on improving the quality of sleep
- It helps in the healing process of stress and trauma
- It improves imagination and creativity.

5. Biofeedback

Biofeedback is a different form of relaxation technique because it involves technology. This technique uses electronic devices that help to monitor a user's bodily sensations, including his blood pressure, heartbeat, body temperature. The thought behind this technique is to give information to the user about his sensations. So, by monitoring a user can control them. There are simpler alternatives of biofeedback techniques, which includes wearable devices, for instance, fitness trackers, chest strap and smartwatch. The person can have a track of all the above-mentioned sensations and can check them after a few hours to analyze what is affecting his breathing or blood rate or blood pressure. In this way, he will become aware of the factors which are influencing and he can also find a way to control them.

6. The Calm Reminder

The calm reminder is a very easy and efficient relaxation technique. You do not need to find a quiet corner to practice this. You can practice it anywhere, anytime. If you want to take a power nap in the office or on the bus. This technique is effective to make you fall asleep in a narrow time.

When your body is tense and it is asking for attention, you just need to think about the word "Calm".

Calm is a composite of four letters: c-a-l-m. Now take each word in order and start the practice.

C = Chest. Calm is the keyword of this technique. In the first step, what you need to do is to breathe. Take longer and deeper breaths. Breathe in from your nose and breathe out from your mouth. With that, relax your shoulders. Loosen the muscles of your shoulder and let them droop. Release the burden from your chest and breathe from your stomach.

A= Arms. The second letter of the keyword calm is A. A stands for loosening your arms, biceps, wrists, hands, and fingers. First, loosen your right arm as you have dropped the heavy luggage and relax your hands and fingers. Then loosen your left arm, with the same thinking.

L =legs. The third letter of the keyword calm is L. L is for legs. Release the tension from your legs, thighs, hips, calves, feet, and toes. Start from your toes and gradually move upward.

M = Mouth. The last letter, M, stands for the mouth. There are multiple muscles from forehead to eyes, from cheeks to lips, from tongue to teeth, and last jaws. Relax your jaw muscles and smile widely to stretch your lips muscles to create tension. Then slowly release the tension and relax your facial muscles.

Keep repeating the word calm in your mind as you are breathing too. This is an instant two minutes relaxation technique to prepare your body and mind for a nap or a little rest.

7. Quiet Ears

Quiet ears are a few minutes and nothing to do with the technique. What you have to do is to:

1. Sit or lie down in a comfortable position.

2. Close your eyes

3. Start taking deep breaths. Breathe in and out from your nose.

4. Place both hands on your head and make sure that none of them is physically disturbed.

5. Bring your thumbs close to your ears and put them in your ear canal.

6. Now you would probably feel a high-pitched sound in your ears as they cannot hear the sounds from surroundings.

7. Listen to this sound and keep your focus on breathing.

8. Do not break the momentum and keep listening to the foundation for 10 to 15 minutes.

9. After completing the time, take your thumbs away from your ears, you will be hearing the sounds more clearly and efficiently.

10. Put your hands at your sides and relax your body now. You can take a good nap after this short-quick sweet relaxation meditation.

8. The Toe Tensing

This is also another quick body relaxation technique.

1. What you have to do is to sit back or lie down.

2. Now close your eyes.

3. Start taking deeper and longer breaths. Inhale from your nose and exhale from your mouth.

4. Start sensing your feet and toes. You might need to remove your shoes if you cannot do this while wearing them.

5. Pull all of your ten toes upward and start to take deeper breaths, while doing this. You have been creating tension in your toes. You can also count to 10 to not get distracted.

6. Now release the tension slowly, first from the right foot and then from the left foot.

7. Let them relax for ten seconds. Repeat this technique again until you feel the calmness in your body.

The technique is useful to draw your tension from your body.

Chapter 6 - Meditation for Self-Love and Inner Peace

We are constantly comparing and judging not only others but our own personalities too. When we see someone more successful than us, we start doubting our capabilities and potential. We see ourselves from the standards that society has set. And when we cannot compete with those standards, when things don't work how we want them, we start hating ourselves. Behind all this, our mind is the one who is letting aloof this happens to us. We are always caught up in a tension between how things are, and how we think they should be, or how we would want them. Our mind's constantly reminding us about our failures, limitations, and shortcomings. There is always inner chatter going on in our minds. Thousands of thoughts regarding how we look, and how we should look, how much we are successful, and how much we should have been successful at this age, are coming into our minds one after the other. And eventually, we become victims of low self-esteem and we have to face adversary repercussions in return. We not only lose our physical health but our mental health also deteriorates severely. We not only stop caring and loving ourselves rather our relationship with other people also gets badly affected. We get anxious thinking about our future and our stress level rapidly expands in certain situations.

We couldn't experience inner peace as our minds are always cluttering and making judgments. But Meditation provides us an environment where we learn to let go of resentment and all the thoughts of self-doubt, and self-hate. Meditation offers us a state, a state of stillness where we feel alive and worthy. A state where all the negative thoughts do not matter for a few minutes and in those moments, we learn to love ourselves that we have long forgotten. Meditation teaches us how we have control. Scientific research has also shown meditation help to improve our sense of self-compassion and self-love.

Meditation makes us aware that fundamentally, all radical change comes from within.

How to practice?

- **Find a serene and silent place to be:** Be in a dignified and relaxed seated position. Or feel free to sit against the wall. You can use a meditation cushion also if you have to. You can be in the sitting position as long as you will not get physically disturbed for the next few minutes or so.

- **Place your hands comfortably in your lap facing upward:** Lengthen up through your spine. keep your shoulders relaxed and slightly roll them back to open your chest a bit more.

- **Once you're seated, gently close your eyes, or soften your gaze:** And begin to breathe in through your nose, then expand your lungs and belly as much as you can and finally breathe out from your mouth slowly with relief. Take another deep breath to make yourself fully relax as you breathe out through your mouth. As you breathe, be fully aware of your mind quality and your body's state. Inhaling is just an act of self-love; pause is to feel the love and exhaling is the outcome of self-love which is relaxation.

- **Pause for a moment to enjoy that feeling of being stopped:** And not thinking about the mind. Just acknowledging the moment of being fully present and still. It is the moment of ultimate freedom. Here your mind is lighter and free from all the thoughts of self-doubt, judgments, and criticism and it is also ready to get flourished by thoughts of positivity, self-loving, self-compassion, and kindness. And if the mind wanders off at any point in this meditation, know that it is completely okay. What you have to do is simply bring back the focus of mind to the breath. And notice how thoughts are coming and going. You have to just observe. You will not segregate the thoughts that this is positive or this thought is negative. You will let thoughts float like clouds in the sky and you are just watching. And just this opportunity to check in with the body.

- **Go for a quick body scan:** Notice if there is a feeling of heaviness or lightness in the body? Notice if there is a feeling of restlessness or stillness? Notice where is the body holding tension? With that, notice where in the body you feel the movement, the rising and falling sensations of the breath. Keep all of your focus on the awareness of your breath and on your bodily movements on inhaling, holding, and exhaling the air.

Now there are two choices for you for your comfort level. Either you want to visualize a picture or you want to affirm a few words to yourself.

- **Loving-kindness visualization:** Imagine yourself sitting, lying somewhere that is a comfortable place. Let go of any inner chatter, let go of any tension in your mind or body and imagine there are warmth and light above your head. A direct ray of sunlight going directly into your body. As it enters, you can feel your body is getting cleansed and all the tension and stiffness is wiping out. The sunlight goes in through your head, moves from the legs to your waist and into your chest, and finally goes down to the toes. As it flows from your body, all the muscles are getting relaxed and feeling lighter. Imagine a point has come, where there is not any kind of discomfort or tension in your body. Your whole body has been radiating with all the feelings of comfort, compassion, kindness, acceptance, and love. Enchant in this feeling of surreal self-compassion and kindness and fully enjoy this moment to the core.

Self-loving and self-acceptance technique

To have self-love and compassion repeat these statements by challenging any time of negative thoughts in your mind.

So, hear yourself saying this.

"With all my faults, weaknesses, and confinement, I want to completely and deeply accept and love myself."

"With all my blessings, ability, and force to love, I want to complete and deeply accept and love myself."

Repeat these phrases to yourself as many times as you want until you feel the lightness and warmth in your body and mind.

Both of the techniques are helpful and practiced widely according to personal preferences. And bring your focus back to breathing.

- **Keep breathing:** And allow yourself to focus on the sounds around you. You might hear the sound of your breath. Or the whizzing of air, or the car passing by, or people's chatter. Just continue to shift from hearing one sound to the other and with focus, you will notice that all the sounds and noise have been transformed into waves of relaxation and calmness in your mind. And whenever you feel complete, just gently open your eyes again.
- **Love:** you have to believe that love is not something to be found, rather this is something that is already inside you. And it got covered by the surface of worries, self-doubt, judgments, negativity, and criticism.
You just have to keep breathing deep and long to wipe the thin surface of these elements and then you will witness the new light and warmth of self-love and care.

And before getting up from the place, just take a moment and notice how your mind feels, and notice how your body feels. You have to neglect any temptation to judge or doubt the meditation you have just practiced. Believe that with only practice, you will get comfortable with this feeling and quality of mind.

The truth is the more we practice this meditation, the more we start to feel these feelings.

Just start with this intention to carry this quality of mind from your meditation into wherever and whatever you are doing next.

How is it helpful?

- This meditation is helpful to release doubtful, judgmental, and critical thoughts from the head.
- This meditation is meant to develop feelings of self-love and compassion in yourself and kindness for others.

Meditation for the Inner Peace

Why are we not able to have inner peace? Why are we not able to reach our maximum potential? To answer these questions, we blame our environment, and our situations and circumstances.

We think that to have inner peace, we need to achieve our goals, and we need to sort all the things from our relationships to our jobs. But this is not the key to have inner peace. There is a very huge possibility that we can experience inner peace even when we are going through lots of challenges in our lives. So first, we need to understand the meaning of inner peace. What is inner peace to you?

Does it mean a quiet place like home where you come after having a stressful day and find an escape from the stresses of life? Does it mean a free place where you can be yourself without any formality or facade? or does it mean a place where your potential is not confined due to certain circumstances? So primarily inner means the mind or the spirit and peace is defined as a state of tranquility, calmness, and quietness. A stilled and stopped place where one is free from the transitory world.

So inner peace is the inclusion of our thoughts and feelings into a state of serenity, harmony, and tranquility. It is considered that, to achieve inner peace or peace of mind we need to find a suitable way to release our emotions and feelings. To achieve inner peace, the technique we will explore in this chapter is "Resting Awareness". This practice asks us to leave everything aside and we do not have to keep our focus on anything rather we just have to be aware of our surroundings.

How to practice?

- **Sit comfortably:** Be in a conducive place where you won't be disturbed for the next ten to fifteen minutes or so. Sit in a comfortable position, if you want to sit on the floor, sit by crossing your legs, bring the right leg over the left leg and right hand over the left hand. Put your both hands in your lap, make your right index finger touch your left thumb. Upright your spine. Sitting in this position is called a peace position.

  And if you want to sit on a chair or sofa, you can. You just have to be in a position to not be get disturbed by any physical discomfort and your blood can circulate freely.

- **Gently close your eyes:** As if you were going to sleep, close them slightly not tightly. If you want to keep them open, it's okay. You don't have to look at anything, just make a soft focus of everything around you. You just have to be comfortable without getting distracted by anything.

- **Take a deep breath:** Keeping your eyes closed or maintaining a soft focus, start taking big, deep breaths. Breathe in through your nose and breathe out through your mouth. Each time you breathe in, just notice how the air passes through your lungs and goes to the middle of your abdomen every time. As you breathe out, notice how your muscles in your body soften. Now, if your eyes are open, gently close them and do this breathing practice a couple of more times.

- **Let everything go:** Allow your thoughts to come and go. You do not have to stop the thoughts. You do not have to change your thoughts. You just have to witness the thoughts without judging them. Just let everything go. All of your worries are related to work, family, the future, and everything else. This technique does not require any effort. You are simply letting go of everything. Just relax every muscle of your body through breathing. Start from relaxing your muscles of the head, down to the muscles of the face and forehead. Relax the muscles of your neck and shoulders. Relax the muscles of your back, chest, and legs, and down to the toes. Notice every part of your body and do not let any part of your body tense or tighten. Try to get a sense of how your body is feeling. Notice whether there is a sense of lightness or heaviness. You just have to notice, not think about it. While noticing your body, also notice the rising and falling sensation of your body as you breathe in and out.

- **It's okay to get swept away with the thoughts:** By doing this meditation, you are not trying to achieve any-thing. So, the mind has to do nothing. So, it is completely fine if the mind gets occupied with any of the thoughts.

You just have to bring it back to have awareness of the surrounding.

- **Nothing to do and nowhere to go:** After settling your body and mind, take a moment and notice the feelings of nothing to do and nowhere to go for the next new minutes. You just enjoy the feeling of having stopped and being still. Start to notice the feeling of weight. How the body is pressed down on the surface beneath you or into the seat of the chair. Notice the sounds around you. Notice if there is any resistance to the sounds. Remind yourself to allow any sounds just to come and go throughout the whole practice. In this practice, you need to change your attention, from noticing your breath to rest in the awareness.

- **Rest in awareness:** You need to let go of any of the focus on the breath now and allow your mind to do whatever it wants to do. Allow your mind to be completely free. Let it be busy and think. What you have to do is to realize that the mind has wandered off. You need to allow the mind to be busy. You are aware of the mind's activity without getting involved in it. Now again, bring your attention back to the rising and falling sensation of the breath for a few moments longer. Let the mind be free again.

This meditation is truly about doing notice, there is no need to focus on anything. You do not have to think about anything. Just let everything come and go. Be aware of your breath, your mind's wandering, your body's rising and falling sensations with the breath, the sounds around you without any resistance or getting involved in these activities. And whenever you feel ready, you can gently open your eyes. Before getting up and starting your daily hassle, just take a moment and notice how it feels in the body and how it feels in the mind.

How is it helpful?

- With this meditation, hopefully, you will find not only inner peace but also you will achieve your sense of limitless potential.
- with a more peaceful and spacious mind, you are not only changing your life but also of those who are around you.

Chapter 7 - Mantras to Obtain Success in Life

We live in a world, where we measure our happiness in terms of being successful and when we don't get success, we start to blame ourselves and become the victim of depression and hopelessness. To avoid such circumstances, we need to change our approach towards the idea of success. Try to bring a change in our life by being more positive and we can do that by adding a few Mantras in our life.

Mantras are the tools that give an object to our mind to focus on. When we keep chanting these mantras in our heads, we are de-cluttering our minds. The mind will not wander off if it has to chant these words continuously. Mantras are a set of a few words which have a divine power to change our life.

Mantras are not meant to be spoken as normal speech. They need to get vibrated from the deep breaths of the lungs. Every mantra has a different vibration which helps us to restore strength and positive energy so that we will be able to deal with any kind of situation in our life. The vibrations help reduce anxiety and minimize stress levels. And chanting them helps to produce positive energy and create a stronger connection between us and our divinity.

There are few mantras, some of them are General and some are from the Sanskrit language. They are considered the most effective mantras to obtain success and happiness in life.

the first of them is;

- **"I cannot do everything today, but I can take one step towards my success"**

Saying this mantra to yourself whenever you are losing hope and doubting your abilities for getting success in your life, calms your nerves and eliminates automatic negative energy in you.

To chant: You need to sit comfortably and take deep, big breaths. Close your eyes and start chanting these words slowly. As you will chant, your breath will get harmonized with the vibration and it will gradually free your mind from all those thoughts of hopelessness and failure. Your mind will wander and will get stuck to the thoughts coming to your head. But what you have to do is simply bring your focus back to repeating these words without being hard on your mind. You have to be gentle and calm during this practice.

- **"I will figure it out"**

Is another very meaningful mantra to do better in your life every day. When you will realize that you cannot be successful in one day rather it is a journey where you will learn from getting failed. What does this mantra mean? It means there will be problems and challenges on the road to success, but you do not have to lose faith. Instead, you need to realize that you are capable of dealing with it "I will figure it out, no matter what". When chanted this mantra with strong belief and devotion will help you take better decisions by throwing the negative thoughts away.

To chant: You can chant this mantra everywhere, it can be your workplace as well. You just have to set your breath and sit in a comfortable position. By closing eyes, start taking deep breaths. Keep your mind on inhaling and exhaling the air from your nose to your mouth. and begin saying these words to yourself in a deep and low voice. Instantly you feel a serene calm in your body. Your mind is busy chanting these words. As you take longer breaths, your bodily sensations are getting calmed and all the thoughts of failing are getting out of your head. As you realize you have been in the right headspace, open your eyes and continue your daily tasks with positive energy in your body.

- **"Om Namah Shivaya"**

Om Namah Shivaya is the most powerful mantra in Hinduism. It is dedicated to their lord Shiva. Before chanting, you need to understand its meaning. So

Om is the sound that stands for the creation of the universe.

Namah stands for showing devotion and adoration to the mighty God.

Shivaya is about the awakening of the inner self.

This mantra is from Hinduism but anyone can bring it into use as it stands for consciousness and inner wisdom.

To chant: You can say these words after waking up or before going to bed. You have to close your eyes and calm your breaths. By breathing in, repeat this mantra over and over again. By doing this your mind will do nothing but to have one focus on repeating this mantra. In this manner your body will be softened as all the stiffness of tension is getting released with the breath. You will continue to repeat, you will be in a transcendental mode or in a state of pure concentration.

- **"Om Vasudhare Svaha"**

This mantra is from Buddhism. It is also called the Buddhist money mantra. It is a prayer to the Bodhisattva of abundance and earth Goddess Vasudhara. Chanting this mantra repeatedly can bring an abundance of wealth, health, or life but this abundance does not mean physical in terms rather it is meant to open your insight.

To chant: It is said that one has to repeat it for more than a hundred to get blessed by the holy deity who will bestow you with abundance. You have to sit in a clean place and give full devotion to the god and goddess. Close your eyes and start chanting these words. Repeat them without getting distracted and within a few minutes, you will see upheaval in your concentration which will lead to the spiritual insight with time.

- **"Jehi Vidhi Hoi Naath Hit Moraa Karahu So Vegi Daas Main Toraa"**

This is the final mantra to obtain success in life. It is chanted when you are not sure of any other success mantra. This mantra means O Lord I am your devotee. I do not know what to do. So do at once whatever is good for me. It is said that this mantra is the final door to success as long as you are saying these with utter faith and reverence.

To chant: the more times this mantra is chanted, the more benefits this mantra will bring. So close your eyes in a clear environment and be fully devoted to this practice and start chanting these words. Your mind will gradually lose all other distractions to get fully concentrated on repeating this mantra. And eventually, you will be able to see a strong faith in being successful in life without any presumptions of getting failed. It will boost the positive energy instantly.

Chapter 8 - Meditation to Energize Awakening

In the world we live, We humans are getting consumed by the sheer pressure and responsibilities. In doing so, we are also risking our mental health and losing our inner peace. The main question is how to nurture peace of mind, compassion, mindfulness, and tranquility? The answer was given hundreds of years ago, that is to turn inward. If we want to discover wisdom and if we want to break the conventional routines to go on a journey to realize our mind's potential. If we want to change our quality of mind, we need to embark on the journey of the inner world. And the more we will go deeper, the more we will observe the change in ourselves. And this unconventional change is called awakening. To explain it in other ways, Awakening is also called having a "Third Eye" or "Inner Eye'. According to Hinduism, the third eye is a door to open higher levels of consciousness and the inner world and since it is not visible it is also called the inner eye. It is present between our eyebrow's junction. And Theosophy sees this awakening in the production of a gland called "Pineal Gland ". The inner eye is considered extremely powerful because it is the source of intuitive and inner wisdom which guides us to develop Insight. It is considered a state of utter enlightenment. Awakening or third eye or inner eye, all these names stand for single conception (but at different places).

Which is to provide us a perception beyond ordinary sight.

Awakening helps us to see clearly and improves our mental quality. It also sharpens our thinking and directs our focus. It also boosts imagination and creativity.

Meditation is the one of few best and simple ways to be awake, and energize awakening.it helps to get rid of all the negative toxins from your mind and body, uses that energy to make us concentrate better.

Awakening meditation, just like any other meditation, demands you to stay put in a calm place.

- **Find a quiet place:** To begin with, start by finding a place quiet enough to let your focus without major distractions. Sit there comfortably atop a chair or on the floor. Set your back up; it needs to be straight. Bring your shoulder down in a relaxed position, and your chest out. Cross your legs before you and rest your open hands on your knees. Your abdominal muscles should be tight to concentrate in meditation. In short, put your body in a place and position, where you would not get distracted physically.
- **Address your mind:** Try to sweep out all types of thoughts from your mind. It is not possible to free your

mind from having thoughts, nor it is possible to stop your mind from thinking. Your mind will not stop to wander or stay quiet. But you can try to not get carried away with the coming thoughts, you can try to not get distracted by those thoughts and if you get drawn by the coming thoughts, what you simply have to do, is to bring your attention back to the meditation gently whenever you realize it. You will criticize yourself because it's the mind's job to constantly think. If a thought lands from nowhere, just acknowledge it and keep your concentration on the object of focus. And we are not yet used to being fully mindful and conscious. With practice, we learn to increase our concentration level. So it is okay to get distracted by the mind, gently bring yourself back to the present and focus on the meditation.

- **Take mindful breaths:** Start taking a bit longer and deeper breaths. Breathe in through your nose and out through your mouth. Make sure, breathing out should take more time than breathing in. and bring your focus on your breath. Notice how your lungs get filled with air. How the breath moves from stomach to chest and finally releases through your mouth. Imagine as you breathe in you are inhaling the quest for wisdom and by holding the breath, you are waking up all the positive energy inside you and when breathing out, imagine you are releasing all the worldly desires, conventions, and tensions out through your mouth.

- **Close your eyes:** If you want to close your eyes at the start of meditation, you can also do that too. What you have to do is to gently close your eyes, and try to be vigilant and present. Don't let your mind get distracted and keep the focus on breathing. And if you want to change your focus on attention, you can bring it to the sounds around you. Don't try to focus on each sound individually, rather just let the sounds come to your ears and don't let them distract you.

- **Time:** Try to meditate for 30 minutes in the least because often, the first 10 to 15 minutes get wasted as we are trying to get rid of all the accumulated thoughts in our mind. The more you will practice, the more you will have the ability and consciousness to avoid any kind of distraction and you will begin to notice some elevated level of consciousness.

If we see meditation to energize awakening from the perspective of Hindu Religion, and what they call it: a third eye, they practice a meditation named **"Trataka"**. This meditation is based on a spiritual belief system that holds the argument that the third eye is right where your six chakras are. And the third eye is a little above the junction of two eyebrows. We need to understand what chakras are? So chakras are energy points in our body that are responsible to bring harmony between our body, mind, and soul. Different chakras have different roles. Six chakras named Ajna essentially help you gain awareness of the surroundings, in a manner that you could start sensing the coming danger and you could perceive things without looking with your two naked eyes. With every session, Chakra shifts your state of awareness and consciousness to higher levels. It also takes away your anxiety and tensions from the core root and transcends into the deeper inner thoughts.

Coming to the technique: Trataka simply means gazing. And if we talk about trataka in the confinement of this awakening meditation, it means gazing to concentrate, and to focus better.

- **Sit on the floor comfortably:** To practice third eye meditation, find a quiet and calm environment to practice and take a sit just like any other meditation, which asks you to sit comfortably. You need to sit in a crossed-legs position on the floor. And if you cannot sit on the floor, you can sit comfortably in a chair, just make sure your spine is erect.

- **Close your eyes and breathe slowly:** Gently close your eyes. Next, start breathing slowly, breathe in through your nose, and breathe out through your nose again three consecutive times. Still, with closed eyes, bring your index finger and thumb together and breathe deep.

- **Third eye and 6th Chakra:** Try to look up your eyes at 20°at at the third eye and 6th chakra that is located just between your eyebrows. You can use your finger to indicate the exact location.

  Draw your eyes towards the junction between your eyes and concentrate on the point and to do so, start to count the numbers from 100 backward to 1. Take two-second breaks after counting one number. Briefly, you have seated on the floor or chair, keeping your spine upright and body relaxed, while your eyes are closed and focused on the junction, and you are breathing slowly and deeply and you are counting numbers backward.

- **The Strain on the eyes:** You probably feel stress and a particular strain on your eyes and this is because you have drawn your eyeballs upwards. The stress is harmless and soon you will get accustomed to it with time and you won't feel the stress.

  Opening of the third eye. A sensation in the middle of eyebrows, signaling that something is happening there. You just have to keep focusing and soon after you begin to see all of your thoughts just like you are in a dream. And then, you will notice a whitish-blue light under the blanket of closed eyes. And this light is the transcendental phase of healing and recovery. Being in this phase, a light will elevate you and you will feel weightless. And you would want to get rid of all the worries and negative thoughts and you just don't want to come out of that concentrated and focused phase. Stay in that position for more than ten to twenty minutes. Now allow yourself to bring your focus back to the sounds around you but still with closed eyes. Give some rest to your eyes. Keep breathing the air in and out. Now, you can open your eyes.

One thing to note: sometimes you may feel warmth around your third eye area while meditating. That warmth can lead to extreme heat and it is a sign of the opening of the third eye. Sometimes irritation could also happen due to intense heat.

Two Accomplishments after Trataka

- Your eyes get exercised and it will make them healthier.
- You learn about focus, the force of intuition.

The First Awakening

There is a technique to open the inner eye, the 1st Awakening. It is about connecting with your soul which is the Pineal Gland. According to Rene Descartes, a famous French Philosopher, this is the place where the soul lives. And this is also a fundamental joining point of the mind and the body. If the gland is already present in our body, then why do we not have mindful insight.? The answer to this question is, we human beings are average beings, living in the realm of the ordinary. And being in the average body, this Pineal gland performs its biological role which is the secretion of melatonin. This hormone is responsible for our sleep. By using appropriate practices, we can reach the realm of higher vision and perception to be called Pineal Gland Awakening or 1st Awakening.

The first stage of 1st Awakening:

- **Sit upright in a quiet place:** Find a calm, quiet place and sit in a comfortable position on the floor by crossing your legs and keeping your spine straight and upright.

- **Inhale air:** Start breathing through your nose and fill your lungs with the inhaled air slowly. Try to hold the air in for the long time you can comfortably hold. And you have to release this air through your mouth but differently.

- **Bring your tongue to the back of your front teeth:** By holding the air in your lungs, prepare your mouth to exhale it. For this, bring the tip of your tongue to the back of your front teeth. You need to make your tongue put some pressure against your teeth as you put to pronounce "th" sound in the word like the, though, then. Now slowly exhale the holding air. As you release the air, your tongue will be making vibrations. The air has been released from the place of connection between tongue and teeth.

- **Sensations and pressure:** After the exhale, your jaw and cheeks are feeling sensations. A particular kind of sensations and these sensations are somehow making pressure and this pressure will lead you to the opening of the eye-inner or third eye.

  It is not one-time practice, you have to repeat the inhaling e and exhaling in a consecutive round manner more than five times at least to create the pressure. This practice will let you register for the expecting experience of opening the inner eye.

The second stage of 1st Awakening:

The second stage of the 1st Awakening is the repetition of the whole procedure of the 1st stage. You have to repeat the process after twenty-four hours. In the due time, your body and mind both will deal with the impact of the first stage. You will repeat the 1st procedure after the first repeat again after twenty-four hours. The second stage is repeating the first stage three times. So, the whole procedure will take three days to complete. After doing this, you have completed the 1st awakening.

The Second awakening starts with the presumption that you have already completed the two stages of the first awakening. You should practice this technique after one week of completing the two stages of the first awakening. This stage is almost similar to the first two stages what you have to do is to:

- **Sit calmly:** Sit in a calm and relaxed position.
- **Breathe deeply:** Breathe in until your lungs get filled and hold your breath for five seconds and breathe out slowly through your mouth. Repeat this three times.
- **Focus on the third eye:** Now bring your focus on the third eye. Deliberately feel the pressure of the eye within you. Keeping your focus on the third eye, start breathing deeply as you did during the first awakening. Breathe in from your nose and breathe out after holding the air in for five seconds, through your mouth with the sound of "May".

The psychic impacts of Awakening

After completing the stages, we will probably have a headache or migraine and if not this, you will sense the pressure in the middle of your forehead and this is the indication of doing practices right. You will notice that the pressure is shifting from one place to the other in your forehead. You probably hear some sounds in your head of what we call "Hearing". With all the physiological occurrences, you will get pretty sure that your inner eye is opening. It is better to practice meditation in the nighttime so your day will not get affected by these things.

After successfully energizing awakening, you will see many changes from physiological to psychic. In physiological transformation, you will go through a shifting pressure in your forehead. You will face a headache or migraine. But these changes are transient. The psychic changes are unending.

- You will begin to learn at a better pace and you will be happy to see an increase in your retention rate of what you learned.
- You will begin to discover your psychic hidden talents
    - **Clairvoyance:** It is to have a clear vision. The ability to have information about a person, object, or event through extrasensory perception.
    - **Clairaudience:** It is the ability to hear which is not present and it is beyond the reach of the ordinary ear.
    - **Clairsentience:** It is the ability to acquire knowledge by the means of feelings.

- The awakening is all about the energy flow of elevated awareness. You will feel the lightness within you.

To energize awakening, this chapter presented three ways of meditation. The first practice was not restricted to the faith of the third eye or inner eye. The second meditation was concerned with the Hindu religion with the belief of having the third eye right between the junction of eyebrows. And the third meditation was aligned with the conviction of the Pineal Gland and its significance as the seat of the soul.

Meditation is a journey of a lifetime and to get benefits from it, we need to practice it regularly. When meditation will be part of your life, you will see the benefits not only when you close your eyes but also when you open them again and go back into your life. Meditation tends to give its benefits gradually. We probably do not see its effects instantly, but after some time when we probably look back and see that we have changed.

Conclusion

So, the primal chore of Meditation is not to provide relaxation rather to make our mind and body a present living, a living being that is free from the uncertainties and peer stress. Being part of a society, there is extreme pressure on our shoulders. We always have to be right, smart, successful, healthy, and we cannot be mistaken, fail, or run at a slow pace. All these expectations and assumptions churn out all our energy and peace.

Our mind is always occupied and fighting with multiple thoughts every moment. And meditation offers it Rest by anchoring its attention to the other objects: it could be breathing, visual imagery, or a wall in front of our eyes. Meditation is a very long and tough path but it is highly enriched with hundreds of advantages like consciousness and mindfulness.

There are as many forms of meditation as many types of health problems are present. We meditate to be more mindful and present by walking or listening to our bodies and the surroundings. We meditate to control anger. We can meditate to be more compassionate and kinder. We meditate to experience inner peace. We meditate to fight any type of anxiety. We meditate to control our blood pressure and heartbeat. We meditate to fight insomnia and have good sleep. We meditate to control our stress levels and to balance our hormone levels. We meditate to be aware of inner wisdom. To be precise, we meditate, our countless problems can get solved by just handling them with acquired tranquility and peace

If we practice meditation daily for only 15 minutes, we can notice positive impacts on our physical and psychological functioning and if we count a few there are enhanced productivity and increased creativity, improved learning and better retention period, improved attention and concentration.

To practice meditation, we do not need fancy clothes or an exotic location. We just need an inclined will and a quiet place to sit. These fifteen minutes can improve our whole day's progress. It carries us more calmly through our day and helps us to control certain medical problems.

To conclude, meditation preaches "the world is in us" and we need to take care of it. But how can we do that? Simply give it time to be still and stop. Giving time to ourselves to relax and enjoy the present moment. Meditation not only helps to purify the mind but also rejuvenates the body. And while meditating, when we bring our five senses into use, we set our all focus now to enjoy it more profoundly and deeply. We purge our mind from all the distressful and detrimental thoughts and we input self-affirming, definite, and positive thoughts. We rejuvenate by relaxing every muscle of the body from head to toe.

An effective and simple rule of thumb is when you opt for meditation and want to make it your part of life, you have to be patient. Because it is a long road and you probably would not witness any fruitful results in your early time but there are long-term benefits of meditating and you will realize after reaching a certain age.